THE
HEALTH
ILLUSION

Is It Killing You?

Dr Sarah Farrant
Award-Winning & Global Best-Selling Author of *The Vital Truth*®

The information in this book is not intended as a substitute for consulting with your chosen health care professional in either of the allopathic, alternative or alternate approaches to health. The author is not responsible for any adverse effects or consequences resulting from the use of any suggestions, approaches or procedures contained in this book.

The Health Illusion: Is it Killing You? © 2014 by Dr Sarah Farrant, DC

The Twister® image on page 128 is owned by Hasbro, Inc. No attempt has been made by the author to own this image. It is used for educational purposes only.

Published by: Vital Wellbeing Ltd

Cover design by: Susie Ward, www.SGWDesign.com

Edited by Jo McKee: jo@jomckee.com

ISBN 978-0-9803185-5-5

To John and Sue Ham, my mum and dad,
for being the perfect teachers.

To Randall, my husband, whose love
is evergreen and unwavering.

To our children: our twins and Anam, Rui and Anais,
thank you for enriching my life with your presence.

To Miss Claire—you changed my life.

~I love you all~

Praise for Dr Sarah and www.VitalMoms.com

'Inspiration for my family ...'

'Dr Sarah has been a source of inspiration for my family and the families that come into our practice. Mums the world over have been crying out for a place where they can go for information, education, resources and support when making responsible health choices for their families. Now more than ever we, as parents, are starting to question the health choices available to us. Many parents are realising that "ignorance is no longer bliss" when it comes to health and they are starting to ask questions. Dr Sarah's book has a simple, clear message about the true nature of healing and health. I am proud to be associated with Vital Moms.'

Donna Moritz, Australia
www.sociallysorted.com

'Transforms you ...'

'Dr Sarah speaks about health but really her interpretation crosses over so many areas of your life. Her dedication to understanding and imparting health and where it comes from will transform you!'

Dr Laurence Tham, Australia
www.laurencetham.com

'Inspiring, unique and life changing interpretation of health'

'The "health" industry is changing rapidly, yet we're still dying at an alarming rate from medical errors and disease. As a result it has become increasingly urgent to listen to a health professional who offers an inspiring, unique and life-changing interpretation of health. Dr Sarah's message is the most sensible place to start.'

Dr Natalie Bird, Australia
www.coconutmybody.com

'Her approach to health is refreshing'

'Dr Sarah's ability to combine her twenty-five years of health industry experience into life-changing insights with practical advice leaves you with many "Ah ha!" moments. Her approach to health is refreshing and her ability to redefine health is ground-breaking. Dr Sarah will genuinely touch and change your life.'

Dr Damian Kristof
www.damiankristof.com

'The voice of reason …'

'What a privilege to sing the praises of one of the world's greatest health leaders, pioneers and visionaries! Dr Sarah Farrant not only cuts to the chase, she cuts through the hype and herd mentality surrounding the health industry. Her message is real, down-to-earth, scientific, holistic, sensitive, intelligent and incredibly honest. She is one of the most inspiring women I know, and someone I often refer to as the voice of reason. Her vitalistic approach to wellbeing is second to none. She is someone who speaks the truth and gives us mothers permission to be the best version of ourselves by trusting our own innate intelligence. What a gift, what a woman. Dr Sarah has changed my life and taught me that an informed mother does know best.'

Kim Morrison
Creator, Twenty8 Chemical-Free Skincare
www.twenty8.com

'The go-to for alternate health …'

'Dr Sarah is the new go-to person for alternate health. Sign up your whole family and get ready to celebrate yourself as the perfect expression of absolute vitality!'

Lyn Olstein, Australia
Primal Therapist

'Sarah gave me what I call an Ah ha!'

'The evening I heard Sarah speak changed many things for me. Her passion, her commitment and clarity gave me passion, commitment and clarity for what she was speaking on and what I knew to be true. I constantly refer to my notes from that evening to help me understand health and wellbeing on a grand scale. I've been speaking about health for the past twenty years but Sarah gave me what I call an Ah ha! A simple message, a different way of saying it and all I had to do was connect the dots and everything fell into place and a new understanding was the result. I've listened to many speakers through out my life but there are very few that give me that Ah ha! Sarah has a quality about her when she speaks which engages you into a world of calm, but at the same time an urgency to take action. It takes a special talent to do that!'

Cyndi O'Meara, Australia
www.changinghabits.com.au

'Not been to a medical doctor ...'

'As the parent of a handicapped child that cannot talk and tell us how he feels, since discovering Dr Sarah we have not been to a medical doctor. If he is not feeling well it is off to our Chiropractor and then after an adjustment, rest and his body will do the healing. The difference in Kameron since beginning this journey has been amazing. We as parents have peace of mind knowing no one is "experimenting" with drug/medical prescriptions on our son. Dr Sarah Farrant has shown us a health approach with no blood and no drugs.'

Caryn, mum, Australia
www.kawanablinds.com.au

'Prompts you to interpret health in a different way'

'We are shaping a world that expects the best possible expression of health. Finding coherent ideas to assist in managing your health is the first step. Dr Sarah uses an engaging speaking style which prompts you to interpret health in a different way. When her message is incorporated into your life you really do begin to see your life unfolding in a very different way. Once you've heard her though there really is no going back! Crossing paths with Dr Sarah and Vital Moms not only changed my life and view on health but also changed the way my entire family thought about health. I can't imagine any other way of living than in this alternate health paradigm.'

Dr Chanelle Rhodes & Dr TomVaughan
www.boostchiropractic.co.nz

'Certainly walks her own talk ...'

'Dr Sarah Farrant is the real deal. She's committed to you knowing the truth about your and your family's health and provides you with valuable information to make informed decisions. Sarah certainly walks her own talk! She's full of energy and vitality and is a true pioneer in the health industry. I'm certainly clearer about my health options. Thank you, Sarah, for your no-nonsense message about health.'

Kay White, UK
www.wayforwardsolutions.com

'You are simply amazing!'

'I loved all your stories and how you live vitalism out in your personal life. You are simply amazing! My practice members raved about your clear and concise method of teaching.'

Bruce Wong, Hawaii, USA
www.lfwchawaii.com

'Incredibly clear in her communication ...'

'By having someone there as a support we have been able to grow and in turn help others to grow as well. Dr Sarah is not only passionate about what she does but incredibly clear in her communication and very importantly, extremely knowledgeable. She is readily available to impart her wisdom. We feel blessed and honoured to have had Dr Sarah enter our lives and know she will continue to have a phenomenal impact on the lives of millions, directly and indirectly! We wish for others that they allow themselves the opportunity to grow and openly embrace the fabulous opportunities that come from Dr Sarah and her wisdom.'

Drs Kelly and Liam McLaughlin, UK
www.dfchiropractic.com

'Pioneering interpretation of health ...'

'If you are looking to change your health then Dr Sarah is the go-to person to help you make the change. Her pioneering interpretation of health and where it comes from will challenge your current health understanding. Dr Sarah arrives ready to awaken you, and break your current health illusions, so get ready!'

Dr Bob Uslander, MD, USA
www.DoctorsOnPurpose.com

'Insightful information has opened my eyes ...'

'You are doing wonderful things for this world by being the shining light of how to live an alternate lifestyle. Your insightful information has opened my eyes to the healthier choices I can make for myself. I believe understanding the difference in health approaches is great knowledge for anyone. Thank you, Dr Farrant!'

Dan Anacker
www.anackerclinics.com

'She's discovered something important ...'

'Dr. Sarah is the rare article. She's discovered something important that we would all do well to heed, about our state of health and optimal well-being. Thing is, she doesn't just teach theory about it, she is a living embodiment of Vitalism and when you meet her you will be compelled by what her life represents—balance and possibilities. I trust Dr Sarah—she's a one-and-only. Get to know her. Your health will thank you.'

Andrea J Lee, Canada
www.andreajlee.com

'Very clear and simple terms ...'

'Dr Sarah's book is a must for people who are ready and open to take responsibility for their health and their lives. It gives us a deep insight in very clear and simple terms of how to take a close look at our inner being. It shows us how to take control of our lives and how to reclaim our power.'

Dr Ben Olstein, Dentist Australia

www.drbenolstein.com.au

'I have a renewed confidence ...'

'Dr Sarah presents a thorough and inspirational perspective of the true nature of our health and the decisions we make with regard to our health. I have been overwhelmed with the numerous, and sometimes opposing options for healthcare that are offered. I have even questioned the decisions I've made to avoid too much intervention. After hearing Dr Farrant speak, I have a renewed confidence in my body's (and my children's) innate ability to heal, in the decisions I have made for myself and my family, and for the future of our health and well-being. Thank you, Dr Farrant for sharing such vital knowledge and encouragement!'

Kelsey Zedwick, USA

'Enjoy the benefits that your whole family is going to achieve ...'

'I want to really encourage you to be a member of Vital Moms. This is such a critical piece of your family's health and wellbeing. It's amazing—you will want to tap in and utilize the resources that are provided for you so you as a mom can make those decisions that are going to best serve your family. So take action, check it out, participate and then enjoy the benefits that your whole family is going to achieve from being a member of Vital Moms!'

Dr Mikell Suzanne Parsons, USA

www.naturalpathfresno.com

'Encouraged me to face unfamiliar territory ...'

'Dr Sarah Farrant played a major role in changing my approach to every facet of life. Yes, that's a big statement. But Sarah has a lot to share! Sarah's example encouraged me to face unfamiliar territory. Dr Farrant's enthusiastic, vibrant leadership demonstrates a new understanding of what health is and how each of us can optimise our own level of holistic growth. If you have been searching for answers from somebody who knows how to live out their own principles in the middle of life's usual demands, you're in the right place.'

Jo McKee, Australia

www.allcourtup.com

'Many "Ah ha" moments …'

'Thank you Dr Sarah for the many "Ah ha" moments during your Vital Health presentation. Armed with so many "Truths" your audience left with a heightened sense of awareness and responsibility not only to their health but that of their families. Thank you for empowering them to now ask the questions!'

Dr Mark Carter, Leeton Australia

'Fresh and pioneering insights …'

'Managing your health really is an extension of your business! If you don't have your health, what do you have? Dr Sarah gives you fresh and pioneering insights into health that will challenge long-held assumptions and free you to make the right choices for yourself and your family.'

Lisa Sasevich, USA
www.LisaSasevich.com

Acknowledgments

This book would have not come to fruition had it not been for meeting my husband, Randall in the early 1990s. The extraordinary journey we have taken together has seen us have many experiences that have helped to shape who we are today. And Randall, for each and every experience—good and bad—I am grateful I had it with you. Thank you for being there to hold my hand, support my crazy ideas, shower me with encouragement and love me for who I am. I love you. Our children Anam, Rui, and Anais who at print are twelve, nine and seven years old and our twins, who passed away prior to us conceiving Anam, form the foundation of most of the stories I have shared in this book. You all teach me and remind me daily of the genius within the human body. You have taught me so much about myself and life. Thank you for the journey we have had thus far and thank you for being the souls you are. It's an absolute pleasure being the one you chose to help navigate your life. I look forward to unfolding the future together.

To Mum and Dad, John and Sue Ham, thank you for being so instrumental in allowing me to think at my own pace in a manner congruent to me; for recognising that I was different to most kids at school. The life lessons you taught me, Dad, on our short drive to school most mornings have never been forgotten; they're firmly etched in my mind and underpin a lot of the stories in some way shared in this book. Although you are not alive to read this book, I believe you will be proud of the contribution I am making to society, specifically health, through the lessons you taught me and the different way in which you encouraged me to look at 'my world'. My hand goes over your heart to say, 'I have the answers inside me, Dad'. Even though I cannot physically touch you anymore and we don't 'see' each other I feel your presence and guidance often. I love you. Mum, thank you for constantly asking me what my contribution was to any situation I was in, whether it is good or bad. You taught me self responsibility, accountability and that I indeed am the captain of my ship; that life is about choice and at every step I get to choose. I love you. Thank you to you and Dad for giving me life.

To Dr Ben and Lyn Olstein, my pillars, your unwavering support of myself, Randall and our children is overwhelming and sincerely appreciated. When times got tough and I wasn't sure how I could continue, a 'text' from you was all I needed to recharge myself and my thoughts to hunker down and continue writing. Thank you for all that you share with me, Randall and our kids. I love you both.

To my mother-in-law Sunday 'Sunny' Farrant ... 'Nana Sunna'. I know there are many people who don't like their mother-in-law but I am not one of them! I have loved you from the first day I met you. Your kindness, your generosity, and your love were showered on me. I am grateful I received you in choosing Randall to be my partner... what a bonus! Thank you for all the times you have unselfishly swooped in to support us while I have headed off somewhere in the world to speak or do a workshop. You are very much appreciated and loved by us all.

To the brain surgeon on the television, thank you for your genius. You changed my life.

To Miss Claire, I loved walking to your little brown door each day. You saw something in me that I didn't see in myself—this hidden gift for systems. You changed my life by simply believing in me and allowing me to be me. Thank you.

To Audrey and Ken Wells, thank you for your friendship and guidance with life and with this book. Your feedback and encouragement has been wonderful and always received at the perfect time.

To Lisa (my sister), Kim (my sister-in-law), Robb and Brad (my brothers-in-law), Cath and Rohan Sutherland (great friends), Ken Parker and Karen Pedley (chiropractors), Mayor of Melbourne Robert Doyle (English tutor), Leanne Picking (Math tutor), Julie Harrison for introducing me to alternative health, Craig for believing in my tennis ability, Reinhold Bartchi (Head of Australian Rowing), Geoff Harris (Co-Founder Flight Centre Ltd), 'The Nanny' for calling CYFS (child youth and family services) and Robyn Wilson (at the time the Ostend medical centre co-coordinator) for the kindness you gave to myself and my children. I thank each of you for contributing to my life in the way you have. I acknowledge that people come into your life for a short time, a long time or a lifetime; either way I am wiser for the experiences I created with each of you and the lessons I've had returned along the way. You have all contributed to shaping the way I view 'my world' and in doing so have helped to shape the stories in this book for others to learn as well. Thank you.

And last but not least I give thanks to all the private clients I have worked with over the years professionally and personally as well as the individuals and parents that are associated with Vital Moms. Thank you for believing in the Vital Moms health and life message.

An important point

My mission is to share the truth about health and where it comes from. As a mum, an educator, a writer, international speaker and founder of Vital Moms I have an opportunity to share the truth—my truth—about health to lessen the noise and the confusion within the health industry. As such everything I have written in this book is my own opinion. The content is my own interpretation which has been accumulated over twenty-five years of health industry experience. I have not been paid by any organisation, person or institution to write this material. I present it to you for educational purposes only. This book (and my opinion) exist to provide you with choice so you can make your own informed decision.

The events that take place in this book are told according to me—Dr Sarah—and the documents written post an event. There are, of course, always two sides to every event; these are stories told from my perspective only.

If you would like to learn more please go to www.VitalMoms. com to find out how you can attend a live event in a city close to you.

And here is the part that 'pains' me to write - if you act on anything I recommend without the supervision of *your own* chosen licensed health professional, you do so at *your own risk*.

Welcome ... come on in!

Each of us is shaped by people, places, things and events in our lives. We draw on the knowledge gained from each of these when making decisions, and it's for us to make the decisions that are right for us. The knowledge I've used when making decisions for my children and for myself is accumulated from over twenty-five years in the health industry, combined with my life experiences, how I was raised and how I've chosen to view my world. I say 'chosen' because I've been very deliberate in creating my worldview.

Not everything is as it seems. We live in a world that is ever-changing; we see what we want to see and our beliefs are shaped by what we are told or what we observe from others around us. Is it true? And how often do you stop to question what you've been told? I was fortunate enough to be birthed to parents who not only taught me the valuable lesson of questioning but also taught me the importance of self responsibility; that indeed my life is my life and I get to experience it in a manner that is congruent to my beliefs and perceptions. The choices I make are a result of these.

To illustrate the contribution a parent can make to a child's life in an exceptionally short period of time, I will share stories of conversations my parents had with me and now the ones I have with my children. As a result of those conversations, I am a life-long learner who constantly wants to understand and know more. However, the more I think I know, the more I realise how little I know. Our family point of difference to others was that my parents taught me about life; they showed me the bigger picture.

I hope, through this book, to give you a transformational moment or two like they had given me. I'd like to show you a new truth; I'd like to give you a new understanding of the human body and health.

I trust that if you are a parent who is losing confidence in the way you approach health that there will be answers for you here. I want to give you hope that your health and life can be different, and give you a sense of trust in that process. I believe in my heart that I have made every attempt to do that by sticking to my vision of *organising the world's health information into bite-sized pieces so people can understand it.* In doing so I have scratched the surface of a complex topic of health which includes the family nucleus. It is my hope that you will want to take a deeper dive into the areas that are pertinent to you. To help you do that I've included additional and free resources at the end of some of the chapters.

In 1934, BJ Palmer said the following:

'IN ENTERING into the study of this book and its work, each should, as far as possible, lay aside for the time being all previous theories, beliefs, teachings, and practices. By so doing you will be saved the trouble of trying, all the way thru, to force "new wine into old bottles". If there is anything, as we proceed, which you do not understand or agree with let it lie passively in your mind until you have studied and gone thru the book for a THIRD time, for many statements that would at first arouse antagonism and discussion will be clear and easily accepted further on, after mature reflection and after repeated understanding. After you have given the book mature deliberation, if you wish to return to your old beliefs and ways of living, you are at perfect liberty to do so …'

And as one of my philosophy teachers, Dr Fred Barge, would say, 'Enuf said!'

Enjoy reading 'The Health Illusion: is it Killing You?'

Health and vitality,
Dr Sarah Farrant
Founder www.VitalMoms.com

Foreword

Quiet desperation

There is a quiet desperation infiltrating the modern world. Our biggest threat to health and life just 100 years ago was infection. But now we are threatened by our body's own immune system attacking itself, causing sickness, disability and death.

Autoimmunity is the term used when the body's immune system cannot distinguish between itself and the enemy. The body has lost its innate intelligence and begins to attack its own tissue, causing diseases such as Hashimoto's, osteoporosis, myocarditis, dementia, arthritis, scleroderma, multiple sclerosis, type 1 diabetes and approximately 200 other known autoimmune diseases.

Not only is autoimmunity an epidemic, but our children are not faring well. There has been a huge spike in the number of cases of autism, Aspergers, ADD, ADHD, allergies and asthma. And once we're in our forties, it's cancer, diabetes and heart disease, or some new rare autoimmune disease. We are desperate for answers.

The answer is out there, but for some reason many health professionals opt for 'wilful blindness' to the detriment of their clients, their family members and themselves. Wilful blindess is a legal term that states that there is information out there that one should know, and must know, but for some reason one chooses not to know. In other words, many people are ignoring the evidence.

Chemicals, excessive birth interventions, abuse of medications, vaccinations, institutionalised and political health care, food additives, modified foods, hydrogenated vegetable oils, genetically modified foods, nano foods, aggressively farmed mono-crops and poor animal husbandry combine to create the rate of sickness we now see, yet our primary care practitioners continue with the mantra of diagnosis and treatment with drugs, chemotherapy or surgery.

The food—or 'food-like substances'—served in our schools, hospitals and retirement homes show utter disrespect that modern political medicine and government has for the intelligence of the human body. Despite our knowledge that food, sleep, sunlight, connection and movement are necessary for the health of the human body, there is a wilful blindness and people do nothing.

But, there is light at the end of a long tunnel. It comes from the whistleblowers who see the disconnect between research and current treatment and paradigms of health care. Whistleblowers are usually seen as slightly crazy and eccentric, but they are in fact passionate about the ideals of their profession and desperately want to do what it right and tell things as they really are. They are visionaries, ahead of their time, with a passion for speaking the truth. They know that if they don't they will have done a disservice to their fellow humans so, despite the consequences, they continue to speak out.

Dr Sarah Farrant is a whistleblower, and this book tells it how it is. If we continue to do the same thing then nothing is going to change and my bet is that it will only get worse. It's time we change the way health (sickness) care is done today. It's time to think differently.

Dr Sarah thinks differently. She articulates the current paradigm and suggests a new one that is not only revolutionary, but evolutionary.

I come from a family that were seen as slightly nuts. In 1960, my father was the 43rd chiropractor in Australia. He was seen as a 'quack' but most people didn't know that his first eight years of work was as a pharmacist. Dad had the advantage of seeing the current paradigm of healthcare (reductionism and mechanism) and was then introduced to a very different way of thinking. The year after my father graduated as a chiropractor, I was born. I was not vaccinated, against the current trend. I was given no medications, prescribed or otherwise. At fifty-four years of age I've never had any form of medication, which most people find amazing and doctors believe is just luck. However, luck played no part. My children also have the advantage of having been given no vaccines or medications, and they're now in their twenties and free of all medications.

Considering that in the western world an average person will take between 40,000 and 46,000 medications before they turn seventy-five, this is remarkable. The difference is that I was taught to think critically and act accordingly.

The current paradigm of health care is based on not listening to the body. A headache, fever or pain is squashed with a pain killer. Infection is destroyed by an antibiotic, taking away the very thing that tells the body it's time to rest, realign, eat simply and slow down.

Current thinking believes the body is inadequate and lacks the capacity to fight infection, cope with pain or birth a baby. As a result, at every stage of life there are outside forces given to a person in order to survive: ultrasounds, vitamin K at birth, oxytocin for the mother, antibiotics, vaccinations, pain killers for those first teeth, booster vaccinations, acne medications, Ritalin, anti-anxiety drugs and, as we age, statins for high cholesterol and radiation and chemotherapy to aggressively treat all cancer. There is an intervention, drug, chemical or operation available at every turn to keep the human body alive.

However, when we learn—and teach our children—about the innate intelligence of the body and that, given the right resources: sunlight, rest, connection, food, clean water and movement, and remove interference to the body's nerve system, then the mind and the body has the capacity to live a full, healthy, happy and creative life.

In order to change we must think and act differently. A revolution is starting that will serve the next generation and this book will propel that revolution. Once you've read it, please don't keep this valuable information to yourself. Inform others and let's start a ripple effect that can change the health of the human species.

Many people revere sportsmen as their heroes. I revere whistleblowers. I watch them and support them, regardless of their industry, because I know that they're not eccentric or crazy—they have refused wilful blindness to tell the truth. They save animals, people, plants and the planet.

Thank you to all the whistleblowers who make a difference in this world.

Thank you, Dr Sarah Farrant.

Cyndi O'Meara,
Nutritionist, author, speaker
Founder of Changing Habits

Contents

How to Use This Book
to Get the Most Out of It

'The journey of a thousand miles begins with the first step.'

— Old proverb

My goal in writing this book was simple …

'To organise the world's health information into bite-sized pieces so people can understand it.'

You will find this book is packed with information to help you navigate the complex and yet simple understanding of health. Unlike my other book *The Vital Truth*® which was a 'dip in' book, this is written in a different way. **Reading it from front to back will serve you best and give you a logical progression of how I have formulated my position.** I'll present tools to help you make an informed decision for yourself and family and an opportunity to connect with who I am. If you feel inclined to 'dip your toes in further' there are questions and resources at the end of the chapters and further resources in the 'About the author' section at the end of the book.

There is a possibility that you could become overwhelmed with the enormity of the changes you would like to make. I suggest pacing yourself; this is not a race but rather an opportunity to take steps towards what is possible in health ... for you and for your child. I certainly do not want you putting this information in the 'too hard basket' or thinking 'that was a nice read' and placing it on the shelf. I would rather you step forward and instigate the changes you would like to make to your life.

It was Einstein who said 'Insanity is doing the same thing over and over again, expecting a different result.' In health, often that different result doesn't come. People remain where they are because they know no different, doing 'it' that way because that's the way it has always been done. Paralysed with fear and unsure of where to go and what the other ways might look like, you decide to stay with what you know, hoping all will be well, popping pills and praying that health will return. Children get 'sicker', lives get messier and before you know it you or your child are on the road to consuming a plethora of medications, ill health and a life of addiction.

I'm here to help reframe for you what health is, to break the illusions that exist around health and assist you with stepping away from the treatment merry-go-round you might be on; doing it *that way* because that is the way it has always been done. My family—myself, my husband Randall and our three children—are living proof of a healthy life outside the 'medicated system' (no medical doctor, no pills, no tablets, no drugs—over the counter or prescribed).

I want you to reclaim your power as a parent who is best positioned to serve your child as he or she grows to make their own choices about health. I want you to have the confidence to make the decisions that are right for your family. There is a simple process to begin making a change. To illustrate this I would like to start where I left off in *The Vital Truth*® with my last chapter on 'Kaizen'.

Kaizen originated in Japan and espouses gradual and continuous improvement. It acknowledges that small, gradual and continual steps are beneficial in instigating and sustaining the change you desire. Change is imminent in our life and every aspect of the change deserves to be acknowledged. Kaizen teaches you to take gradual and simple steps to 'see' the change you want. As the old proverb says 'The journey of a thousand miles begins with the first step.'

As you read, make notes about each chapter. Get the 'extra resources' and complete the exercises to keep you moving. When you have finished, grab a large sheet of paper and write down what you want to change. Once all your notes are organised into one place you'll start to see where your 'first step' can be taken—where is that path of least resistance that will catapult you on your way? Remember you are only looking for ONE place to start ... and then start. It doesn't matter where that is. You can choose to embrace this new understanding of health or you can choose to continue as you have always done, remembering what Einstein said about 'insanity'. The choice is yours.

CHAPTER 1

'Dumb, Dyslexic, and a Dunce'

*'No one is dumb who is curious. The people who don't
ask questions remain clueless throughout their lives.'*

—— Neil deGrasse Tyson

Two visions shaped me.

The first? In 1972 my father brought the family a black and white TV; an electrical item that changed how we interacted as a family. I thought we were rich. My parents were now able to watch the news and variety shows like 'Australia's Bandstand' and my sister and I got to explore the back of the TV, wondering where all the little people lived, calling some of them by name to entice them to come out. The Summer Olympic Games in Munich were being broadcast and I remember as a young five-year-old watching closely as the athletes marched out, goose pimples covering my body at the thought of marching and proudly wearing the Australian green and gold.

Two things happened as a result of watching the Munich Olympic Games: (1) I became transfixed on the greatness of the human body and its muscles, obsessed with 'its' ability to perform, set records and achieve success and (2) I made up my mind to be an athlete and represent Australia at the Olympic Games. In what year this would happen I wasn't clear on *and* the sport was yet to be determined.

Second?

A few months after the Olympic Games had finished, Mum had the TV on while I was preparing the table for dinner. Dad had just got home and my sister was helping Mum get the dinner. A 'news flash' came across the TV. We stopped what we were doing, went to the couch, and Dad turned up the volume. Out came a surgeon dressed in his 'greens' with a mask hanging from around his neck. He sat with a microphone poised in front of him and leant forward, a cue for the journalists who began firing questions all at the same time. The surgeon began discussing the brain surgery he had performed—a first for his time. He spoke of the person being in critical condition but the surgery being a success. I was transfixed on how he could open a person up, look inside, tweak what need to be tweaked (according to him) and close the person back up. Amazed, I wanted to be able to look inside the human body just like that surgeon and 'see' what was going on. As the interview came to a conclusion and my dad got up to switch off the TV, I announced to the family my 'other vision' … 'I'm going to be a doctor and change people's lives.' Secretly, I wanted to be a brain surgeon. My parents smiled, patted me on my back, and we made our way to the dinner table.

That vision was sidetracked …

At school I was constantly challenged. I had created dyslexia— no, I didn't 'get' dyslexia nor was I born that way; it was something *I created* and to this day has been a wonderful gift; not a struggle. The only time I struggled was when I was forced into a system of understanding and learning that didn't support my way of thinking. Unfortunately that labeled me dumb, dyslexic and a dunce.

Each day, and sometimes twice a day, I would be called out in front of the class. 'Sarah, it's time for you to go to Miss Claire.' Everyone knew who Miss Claire was. I walked to her little brown door day after day for almost the whole of my school life. Miss Claire was so patient, gentle and loving with me as I struggled my way through learning to tell the time, read, and comprehend a world according to others. She took the time to allow me to interpret the world *according to me* which included my systems mind and seeing what others don't see.

It was on those trips to Miss Claire that I got to confirm to myself and affirm to the Universe that 'I will be a doctor and change people's lives.' I created a system to say my mantra so I wouldn't miss a day. As soon as I approached the oval and my left foot touched the green grass I would bow my head and begin saying out loud *I will be a doctor and change people's lives* over and over again as I bee lined for Miss Claire's little brown door.

I never gave up on my vision of one day being a doctor and changing people's lives.

Even though I was academically challenged, I loved to study. I loved to work out new ways to look at 'things' and invent new ways to do things—situations, theories, truths, processes, philosophy, words—my systems mind always running. By the later stages of school I lacked a lot of self confidence but I never gave up hope of one day becoming a doctor and changing people's lives. I only knew of one type of doctor back then: medical doctors. We had a lineage of them in our family so I was familiar with the hoops one needed to go through in order to become one.

Tennis was my relief after the academics of school. I would go to my grandparent's house in Kooyong almost every night and train with Craig, my private tennis coach, learning the skill and art of playing the game. I loved learning. I loved being taught; I loved what tennis gave me. I remember my dad asking the principal of the school at the time for 'a dispensation card' to play in the All Schools Tennis Tournament as no child was allowed to have the day off to play in the tournament. I didn't feel game ready, however Dad and Craig thought I was. Mrs St Leon granted me the day off from school—I believe she knew that I was learning about life through my sport. I went to the All Schools tournament and got flogged; I won my first round and was pipped in the second round. Dad and Craig were still optimistic about my skill and ability; I wasn't so sure.

A few months later Craig said 'I believe you are ready for Junior Wimbledon.' I didn't. I remember riding in the school bus to Yarringal on a Year Six school camp at the ripe age of ten. I was sitting in the seat, close to the window and in confidence telling my 'friends' that Craig thought I was ready for Junior Wimbledon. They were all in awe of me attending such a prestigious event. However, it wasn't long after I returned from camp that Craig arrived at training and said he was moving to Germany; he'd accepted a coaching position. That was it for me; I didn't pick up a racquet after that. To this day I am unsure why, with all of my dad's life lessons at the time, I didn't understand that 'when one door closes, another door opens'. I simply lacked belief in myself.

The Caltex Motel ... a life changing moment

My grandparents had a farm at Bega and we used to go to it each school holidays along with my six cousins and my aunts and uncles. Dad bought a cheap large silver metal caravan that we placed on the farm near the tractor sheds. Inside it was a bright pink colour and I mean bright pink! My grandparents had built a huge house on the farm in which my cousins would stay, however Dad, like me, preferred to have his space and stay in another location on the farm.

One year during the drive to Bega, Mum and Dad decided to stay the night at our 'local' motel where we usually stopped to get a bite to eat and stretch our legs. As Dad and Mum brought things from the car, Lisa and I raced around the motel room, deciding where we would sleep, looking in the bathroom, jumping on the beds and opening the drawers. Mum and Lisa then went to organise some food and Dad returned to the car to collect our suitcases. Alone in the room, I opened one of the drawers of the bedside table and noticed a book in it.

I sat on the edge of the bed and opened the book. I wondered why the book was separated into columns down the middle with words on either side and numbers at the beginning of paragraphs. I had never seen one before and was fascinated. I loved books; I loved being surrounded by them, staring at them and holding them, even though I couldn't read them. As I sat flicking through the pages, Dad walked in with a suitcase in each hand. He glanced at me, promptly placed the suitcases down against the wall and said, 'Close the book and put it back in the drawer.' As he walked towards me he looked directly into my eyes with an air of understanding. I did as I was told and closed the book, popping it back in the bedside table draw. He knelt down in front of me, placed his hand over my heart and with absolute certainty, confidence and knowing said, 'Sarah you have all the answers inside of you. All you have to do is ask the question and trust your answer.'

My life ... in an instant ... was changed *forever.*

CHAPTER 2

Blinkers On—Blinkers Off

"Hold the vision, trust the process.'
— author unknown

The giant vision board!

As a young girl I remember people and friends walking into my room and asking what colour the walls were because you literally couldn't see any paint! I had posters of athletes on my wall ... *everywhere.* Fortunately for me, Roger Gould—*the* tennis photographer of the day—was a good friend of my parents and would sometimes give me a 'real' photo of one of the tennis players. Mum also bought me yearly subscriptions to 'Australian Tennis'. I wouldn't read the magazine because I was so challenged with reading, however I would scour it for images that I could place on my wall.

The images were specific and they had to demonstrate power, strength, athletic ability and FOCUS. I had to be able to 'see' the muscles working. My room was one giant vision board! I wanted to have muscles like the players I was staring at every night while I drifted to sleep; I wanted to be like every one of them. At nine years old, I'd begun to interpret health being about fitness and what you looked like.

At school I excelled at physical education (PE) class. I was the 'top dog'; it didn't matter what sport we were doing—I played to win. I had a surge of confidence every time PE class came around. As I neared the end of my school life I was asked the standard question, 'What do you want to do after school?' It's a pathetic question when you've only been alive for sixteen years, never seen the world, let alone explored your own community, or never had an opportunity to experience different careers because you're inside an institution. Weird. Anyway, my reply was always, without fail 'something to do with the human body and sport, probably a PE teacher.' Most agreed that I would be best suited to doing this 'line of work'.

But, secretly … I wanted to be a doctor.

I remember at twenty-one sitting in the formal lounge room at my parents' house and my uncle, a medical doctor, asked me what I wanted to do with the rest of my life (I thought life had only just begun). I said I want to work with women and children because women will always be having children. I was thinking personal trainer or fitness coach, something along that vein. My thoughts were steering me in the correct direction.

I went through Year Twelve at a time when the whole year's work was tested in one exam. Your possible top score for any subject was 100% and, regardless of what you got for your other subjects, if you didn't pass English with a minimum score of 50%, you failed your HSC. English was my Achilles heel, so Mum and Dad organised an English tutor in my last year of school. They chose my English teacher, Mr Robert Doyle, who went onto become the leader of the Victorian opposition and the Lord Mayor of Melbourne. Mr Doyle knew it wasn't easy for me but he believed in me and gave me the strength to believe in myself. I have this wonderful visual of him standing near our front door, speaking to me and my mother with his intense eyes, sharing words of wisdom after my final tutoring session with him. I'm eternally grateful for what he did for me.

I struggled with the books we had to read for the English exam and my comprehension was still very limited at this older age. Thankfully Mum found a company that printed 'summary books' of the books we were meant to read for the English exam. She bought one of each. I found I could understand these books because someone had taken the time to organise the content which stimulated my systems and visual mind. I passed English with a score of 51 and was so relieved, but I failed Biology with a score of 49. Suddenly I was at a loss as to what I would do as I was well off the marks to get into PE college. My parents, however, were pleased because I received an overall pass and they acknowledged that night how difficult the whole of my school life had been.

During my later years at school I had switched my sport focus from tennis to rowing. Actually I was in Form Two (Year Eight) when I went and begged Miss Gell, my PE teacher to let me row. I touted that my father had been a rower, as well as my uncle, and my grandfather Basil had been a rower and later a state (Victorian) champion as well as an Australian record holder for the mile back in 1930s—and as such, I should be allowed to row! Unfortunately she didn't see it my way. However my persistence eventually wore Miss Gell down. I was allowed to get in a boat.

I loved rowing and the feeling of freedom while on the Yarra River. I would train hard during my sessions with not a worry to be had over my school work. In fact my first ever trophy (not medal!) came from rowing; everyone at the school was surprised, but none more than us. The school had no rowing facilities. In fact we had no rowing program. Those of us who rowed simply loved it. The school rented old, very wide, very heavy wooden boats from Scotch College, a local all boys' school a few suburbs away. The school was so impressed with our victory that our trophies were awarded to us one morning in school assembly.

When I completed school and didn't get in to what I wanted to I continued to row and, as soon as the HSC exams were over, became a member of the Melbourne University Rowing Club down on the Yarra River in Melbourne. You didn't have to be a Melbourne University student to row for them. I would train up to four times a week and race every weekend, always coming home with a bag full of trophies. I soon became obsessed with wanting to compete for my country in rowing, and matching that to my vision as a four-year-old watching the Olympic Games and saying to myself 'One day I will be wearing the green and gold at an Olympic games.' I realised early on that I was way too slight to compete in the heavyweight division (those ladies are tall and larger than I could ever get to) and I was too small to compete as a lightweight, so I asked myself how I could fulfill my vision of wanting to go to the Olympic Games. I decided to become a coxswain, thinking my strategic and systems mind would be of use. A year after making that decision I just missed the national team by a smidgeon. I returned home from Tasmania where the nationals were held, rather dejected and wondering what else to do with my life. I continued to train at Melbourne University Rowing Club, running and cycling every day. Then, on a Thursday afternoon, the phone rang. On the end of the line was Simon Gillett, a national rowing selector at the time.

'Hi Sarah, this is Simon.'

'Hi Simon.'

'I'm calling to offer you a place in the Australian Rowing team as coxswain of our heavyweight team. Would you like to accept the place?'

I began to shake uncontrollably and replied 'Are you serious, Simon, or is this a prank?'

'This is no prank Sarah.'

'I've been waiting for this day my whole life!' I said. 'I accept!'

I had to be at the Australian Institute of Sport (AIS) in Canberra, ACT on Sunday. It was Thursday when Simon called me. I hung up the phone and buried my head in my hands. Tears began to well as I realised the day of selection had arrived. I let the tears flow and then yelled out to Mum the good news. Mum was so excited, congratulating and hugging me and then went into organization mode … *right what do you need to get?* While Mum was getting a list sorted I called Dad's direct line at work.

'John Ham.'

'Hi Dad, it's Sarah.'

'Hello Sarah. To what do I owe the pleasure of this call?' as he would say each time I called him.

'I just received a phone call, Dad, from Simon Gillett. He offered me a place in the Australian Rowing Team!' Tears began to well in my eyes as silence hit the line. I knew Dad's eyes were filling too, proud of what I had accomplished and a vision that had come to fruition. As he cleared his throat he asked, 'When do you have to be there?'

'This Sunday!'

'Well you'd better get packing!'

Sunday came around fast and before I knew it I had finished packing my car and was about to embark on a life-long dream to represent my country in my chosen sport of rowing. To win gold at the Olympic Games became my vision; it was all that mattered. My middle name became 'focus'; nothing else mattered in my life except training and wanting to win every competition we entered. I lived a portion of each year at the AIS for three years before my 'fate day', as I call it, arrived.

Despite the ups and downs of making weight and the mental challenges of managing a team with decidedly different personalities I enjoyed my time at the AIS, however my departure—my 'fate day'—was far from happy. We were heading into our pre-regatta racing before competing overseas. I was called into the head coach's office for a discussion yet again on my weight. I always seemed to have 1 to 2 kg to lose to make the 45 kg limit. We were four weeks out and the head coach, Reinhold Batschi, gave me the ultimatum: 'Lose the weight by the regatta or you're out!'

As the time got closer I remember going downstairs and outside into the concrete corridors of the AIS dormitory quadrangle. I made a reverse call to my parents; my devastated voice said it all. Hearing Mum's voice was enough to release the months and months of pent-up tears. Through my muffled sounds I said 'I've had enough, no more. I'm resigning from the team. I want to come home.' My mum, never one to solve a problem for me and constantly teaching me to trust myself said 'Are you sure this is what you want to do?'

'I am sure.'

Once I resigned from the Australian rowing team I had no idea of what I wanted to do other than it had to do with the human body, sport and fitness. Yet, literally the day after I resigned feeling dejected, unwanted and discarded, I went to the mail room at the AIS to collect my letters. There was a letter in there from The Australian College of Physical Education (ACPE) in NSW. I thought 'That's odd,' and opened the letter. Inside was a cover letter from the principle inviting elite athletes to apply to the college for a place in the physical education teaching program. I could not believe what I was reading. This was a specialist college which understood that elite athletes were not necessarily focused on school work as much as they were on their chosen sport, and as a result athletes could study physical education while finding support for their training. Entry was based on your sporting performance, your level of achievement within that sport and having passed your last year of school. What score you got didn't matter.

I called Dad and Mum and told them about the letter I had received from ACPE. They were as stunned as I was. I said I would like to investigate it more and mentioned it was a private college. Dad and Mum both said they would pay for my tertiary education—only one—if I wanted to go and study rather than going immediately from rowing to the work force.

I made a few phone calls and before we knew it Mum, Dad and I were sitting in the principal's office having an interview. A few weeks later I was offered a place in the program. I didn't even move back to Melbourne; I simply went straight from Canberra to Sydney. I lived in Lane Cove for most of my time and loved going to college every day to learn about the human body, health and different sports. I passed all my subjects with As and Bs, proving to myself that you excel in things and subjects that you LOVE!

During my study I worked as an aerobics instructor, building up a big following on a Tuesday and Thursday evening in Strathmore near where the college was. Besides taking the classes I spent a lot of time teaching my students about health and nutrition. I taught health was about how you feel, and if signs and symptoms were present then the body was sick and you had to treat it. I used to struggle with this thought process as the experience I'd had with my own body and the trust my parents had taught me seemed to go against this interpretation. However I didn't think much of it and carried on teaching the 'sickness and treatment' paradigm of health.

After graduating ACPE I travelled for over six months around the USA. I returned to Melbourne, my home city, to assist my best friend Cath, who I had studied with at ACPE, establish Australia's first gymnasium within a shopping centre. We wrote the systems and implemented the ideas. I soon became an instructor at the gym and began to build up my own private clientele. I also began my own business training elite athletes outside of the gym and quickly got a name for myself in the strength and conditioning world: working with national basketball players, world aerobics champions and touch football players. Ironically I found myself back at the AIS lecturing to sports groups about talent identification, how to find the people and what to look for. I was invited not long after that to speak at the first national strength and conditioning conference but turned it down, I didn't feel ready to stand on a stage and speak! I noticed with all the athletes I trained and mentored that there was a missing piece to their preparation—the mental understanding of themselves and their belief in their ability. They lacked an ability to see themselves performing in the way they wanted to. This ignited an interest in sports psychology which had just taken off while I was studying at ACPE.

I got into triathlons while I was working at the gym. Each year Cath and I would register to do the BRW series, as it was called then. It was during this time that I had the bright idea to establish Australia's first triathlon club within a gymnasium, so Cath and I did. The gym was called 'The Winning Edge' and in those days words were beginning to be printed on the back of the Speedo bottoms (swimming gear) so logically we decided to run with 'wedge' on ours!

During this time I turned to playing touch football. I was selected for both the Victorian team and the Victorian country team. However, I slowly began to not enjoy sport—participating, watching it and mentoring in it. I was confused with my life and where I was going; I was burnt out. So, in my mid twenties, I took myself off each week to see a psychiatrist to chat about my life. I saw him for two years and learnt so much about myself during this time, and not once was I ever offered medications. I wanted to step away from all things sport, however my challenge was that sport had defined me and the thought of not having sport in my life was daunting. I felt lost. I resigned from the gym, told my private clients that I was not going to be coaching anymore, stopped all work and went on the dole (government assisted living) to find 'me'; to understand who I was when I wasn't being defined by either playing sport or mentoring those in it.

I turned to my second love …

I thought about traveling, however I needed money to do that. I'd also met a wonderful man called Randall and didn't want to leave him. So I decided to do the next best thing and apply to Flight Centre Ltd for a position as a consultant. If I can't fly I might as well help people organise their trips. I went through the interview process and within a few weeks was offered a position. I adapted to the systems rapidly simply because of my systems mind. However, mastering the systems quickly and making good money meant that I was bored very quickly. I needed something to stimulate my mind and I decided the missing piece was psychology. So I applied to La Trobe University's Psychology program in Melbourne. At the same time that I applied to La Trobe, a job posting was advertised via the morning faxes from Flight Centre's head office. Head office was looking for a person to fill the role as part time personnel manager for Victoria. 'Perfect,' I told myself. 'I can fit it in around my psychology study.' I was speaking to myself as if I already had both!

I applied and went to the interviews—psychology and personnel manager—and I got both. Suddenly I was shot into head office with 66 store managers underneath me and 386 staff that in some way I was responsible for. I felt out of my depth but certain that I could fulfill the role. I simply went back to my systems mind. I placed advertisements, culled the applications, scheduled the interviews and then sat interviewing the people, one on one.

After a few months of doing this I was bored out of my brain! I'd mastered another system and now wanted to change it. I worked out what it was costing Flight Centre Ltd, bearing in mind that I was representing all five of their brands at the time: Flight Centre, Great Holiday Escapes, 24 Hours, Student Flights and Corporate Travel. I named it 'the vacancy rate' and it came to a multi-million dollar figure. The way recruitment into the company was being done was archaic compared to the rate at which the company was expanding. There had to be a new system to match the expansion. The thought of designing a new system helped to keep me stimulated in what quickly became a really 'boring job'.

My mantra after every one-on-one interview became 'There has to be a more efficient way to recruit people into the company!' At times I was putting in twelve-hour days and only seeing fifteen people. It seemed insane. I made it my mission to help this company fulfill its vision of global expansion at the rate it wanted to accomplish it. I picked up the phone and spoke to dozens of different people, asking them in-depth questions about their recruitment process. There was one call that changed it all for me. The person said 'group interview' and I was sold. That was it: let's get as many people as we can into a room and mass recruit. Managers could have autonomy over selection so I would no longer receive complaints with regards to the person I had sent them. I was excited at the thought of filling a room with people and welcoming them to the company. The only problem was there were barely any companies using group interviews at the time so I had to invent a whole new model to fit with our Flight Centre way of doing business. It was the mid 1990s and I had a blank canvas to make my own.

I set about investigating companies that were doing group interviews and skipped many a psychology class at times to go and speak with people about their process. Once I had enough of an understanding I began to write it, tweaking certain things here and there. When I was happy with the process *and* I could visualize it really clearly in my mind I made up booklets with a picture of a round world map on the front, named the cover 'Group Interview Process' and rolled it out at a Monday morning meeting to Geoff Harris—one of the owners of the company—and other significant people at head office. It was a no-brainer and a win-win for company induction and expansion. All bases were covered, I just had to do a good job at delivering it to the 'powers that be' around the table.

At the end of the meeting Geoff said 'Let's trial it.'

'Awesome,' I said. 'I'll get the first one organised.'

Within four months Geoff called a meeting with everyone at head office. He announced that positions were going to be terminated as the company began to rationalize. It was my turn to be called. Within minutes of sitting down he said 'We're letting you go.' A nice way of saying 'You're sacked!"

I left not knowing why, and still to this day don't know, other than knowing I did what I needed to do to assist with getting a system up-to-date to match a company's global vision and did so very successfully. Essentially I had worked my way out of a job because this process could run itself. The 'group interview' is still used today as a recruitment vehicle and I smile each time I walk past a store at the thought that perhaps the person behind the desk come into the company via the process I created.

I walked out of Flight Centre not bitter but, rather, complete. I did what I needed to do. While I was at Flight Centre and completing my psychology course a husband and wife came into our life. They were chiropractors. I used to see Karen and Randall used to see Ken. We had been receiving regular weekly adjustments for about a year and I noticed I slowly began to form this new way of looking at the body due to their subtle education. I began to interpret health in a different way. I certainly couldn't define it back then but I knew there were changes taking place in how I was thinking.

No longer did I believe health was about how you felt, but what I thought it was instead, I could not tell you. I owe so much to Ken and Karen for slowly but surely bringing me back to my love of the human body and health.

Entering into a new understanding of health …

I was amazed with what chiropractic was and the opportunity it afforded me to see health differently. I quietly began to research chiropractic and education. At the time Randall was working as a Grade Six teacher at Glamorgan in Toorak, the junior campus of the prestigious Geelong Grammar. They had internet access so after work I would go to Glamorgan to meet Randall and while he did extra work and class prep I would sit on his computer and research chiropractic.

At our next appointment Ken and Karen told us they were moving to Tasmania, Karen's home state. They wanted to celebrate and asked if we would like to join them along with two other couples for dinner. Of course we said 'Yes!' It was at the dinner that a life-defining moment occurred. I asked Ken, 'If you had the chance to study again, where would you go?

'Palmer College of Chiropractic.'

The next day I went to La Trobe University and spent the morning exploring chiropractic on the computers in the library. The internet was only a recent addition to the organisation of information and Palmer College of Chiropractic (Palmer) had a very rudimentary website. I printed off all the information I could—which was the whole of the website —there was no cut and paste back then! I stapled the wad of paper together and went outside..

Sitting on the step outside the union building, I read::

'Health is physical, chemical and emotional wellbeing and not necessarily the absence of disease of infirmity.'

'The nerve system—brain, spinal cord—is the master communicating system.'

'You are a self-healing, self-regulating organism that is constantly adapting to your environment.'

And ... in the top right hand corner it said 'Click here for Doctor of Chiropractic program.'

'Doctor of Chiropractic program ... what?' I said to myself.

Nerve SYSTEM brain spinal cord ... DOCTOR. I began to cry, tears flowing everywhere, unstoppable, students asking if I was okay. 'All is perfect,' I said. I brought forth for the first time in years my hidden four-year-old little girl saying to her parents, 'I will be a doctor and change people's lives.' The only doctors I knew of were medical ones; how wrong I was.

I drove home late that afternoon from La Trobe with tears still rolling down my eyes, wishing someone had invented wipers just for your eyes. I knew in my heart this was 'it': this is what I had been waiting to find all these years since retiring from rowing. Now it was presented in front of me and I didn't want to miss the opportunity.

There was only one problem … my husband.

We had just got married, just bought a house and just bought a new car. How was I going to tell him?

As I walked in the door Randall was making dinner. I had the wad of paper tucked close into my left arm. There were no tears, however my eyes felt red and sore. He noticed the redness.

'What's wrong?'

'Nothing' I said, 'Everything is perfect … that's the problem.'

I placed the wad of paper on the kitchen bench and with absolute certainty said, 'I'm moving to America.'

His jaw dropped. 'You're what?'

'I'm moving to America. We can do one of three things: you can come with me, you can stay and we can have a long distance relationship or we can get divorced. I'm fine with whichever one you choose,' my voice became distant as I walked up the hall to hang up my jacket. I was so clear I was to go to the USA and study. Randall wasn't so sure and took another three months to make up his mind. In the meantime I had done the application for him as well.

One night he said 'Yes, I want to study,' and before he knew it I was selling our car, organising with Cath my friend to have a Camberwell market stall to sell 'stuff', organising a place to stay with an Aussie student in the USA when we arrived and speaking to real estate agents to decide whether to rent our house or sell it. It was a mammoth move. Our parents, of course, thought we were hare-brained idiots and utterly stupid to throw away 'good jobs', forgetting that I didn't even have a permanent one. At the time I was locuming for travel agencies and had just completed psychology.

We knew it would be a scary and yet fabulous decision. In the end we sold everything we owned except for a few boxes which we stored in Cath and Rohan's attic. We simply needed the finances to fund the study.

When we arrived in the USA we looked for a place to live immediately as we were staying for only a week with Trevor, the Australian studying at Palmer who I'd found via the 'Palmer grapevine'. We found an unfurnished apartment, took it for six months and promptly began to look for a house to buy. Houses were cheap over there and with money in hand from the sale of our home in Australia we had some cash for a deposit.

We found a house, put a $3,000 deposit on it, and rented out the other half which paid the mortgage and enabled us to live bill-free as well. We worked five jobs between us to make additional ends meet and applied for academic scholarships which Randall on numerous occasion was the recipient of. We too were the first married couple to ever receive independently the largest endowed financial scholarship in chiropractic—the Vogt Leadership Scholarship—in recognition of future leaders in the profession. We also made a massive, colourful chart on each of the cranial nerves that we sold. It is still being sold at the college and all funds go to helping military veterans fund their education.

I remember my first philosophy class was with Kiwi-born Dr Maxine McMullin, considered the pioneer of pediatric chiropractic. She spoke about Above-Down-Inside-Out (ADIO) and Innate Intelligence. I loved what she was saying and chased her after class down the corridor to ask more questions. She said, 'Come to my office and we can chat some more.'

I started walking with Maxine to her room, yelling to Randall 'I'll meet you on the skywalk in thirty minutes.' Little did I know that it would be at least an hour later. I found Randall sitting on the side ledge in the skywalk waiting patiently. I approached him with my red, sore eyes and he immediately knew I had been crying. I placed my bag down and plonked beside him.

Are you okay?' he said as he wrapped his arm around me.

Tears welled more and more I said 'I feel torn and ripped apart; everything I knew and had been taught about health to this day I feel is not true.' I was dumbfounded, in disbelief at what Maxine had shared; it made so much sense. My head was spinning and my world as I knew it was shattered.

My blinkers were off.

 Ah ha!

* Life is not as it may seem.
* Everything you know to be true can change in a split second if you're open to learning.
* Listen to the whispers pulling you in a certain direction.

CHAPTER 3

Pivotal Changes

'Ask any successful person to look back over the events of his or her life,
and chances are there'll be a turning point of one kind or another.'

—— Bill Ranic

In 2008 I mapped my life and I have to say I loved it. I hadn't done it before and it was fascinating to do. I noticed the *pivotal changes*—highs and lows—and how each interacted with the one before and after it; doors closing and opening. There were three pivotal changes as I've journeyed through my life that have been influential in 'nudging me toward the view on life that I take today. All three assisted me in how I now choose to parent and educate my own children and the thousands of individuals and families who are associated with Vital Moms.

My first pivotal change took place when Dad said 'Sarah, you have all the answers inside of you. All you have to do is ask the question and trust the answer.' Dad was a Socratic father choosing to use systematic, disciplined, deep questioning to allow me to reach my own conclusion. It was very frustrating as a young girl not having anyone to solve my problems for me, answer my questions or help me make a decision! My questions to Dad were more often than not bounced back with another question until I would reach the conclusion myself or walk away in absolute frustration because there he was again asking question after question after question. Argh!

However, I learnt that *what I think I don't know I actually do know.* It was a powerful parenting style and very forward-thinking of Dad to do back in the '70s and '80s. I use Dad's teaching with my children and the people around the world who I mentor. The good news is that if I can learn it, so can you.

At the age of ten I tested what I was taught at age seven by Dad. My mum was making some biscuits (cookies) in the kitchen and I was doing my homework in my room. I could smell the aroma drifting around to my room so I thought I would go and investigate—perhaps even lick a beater! I raced around to the kitchen and Mum had almost completed the mixing. I asked about the type of biscuit, the ingredients and then asked if I could lick the beater. 'No, you can't!' I then coughed a few times and you would have thought Mount Vesuvius was erupting in the house. Mum switched off the beater, grabbed her car keys, raced to the closet and grabbed a blanket, bundled me up, and took me to the car. We took off at what felt like breakneck speed driving up the road to Uncle Richard, our family medical doctor. I remember staring out the window, the rain pouring down and asking Mum 'Why are we going to Uncle Richard? He'll only write another prescription for amoxicillin.'

'Well, I don't want your cough to get any worse.'

We headed into the surgery and because of our family connection were taken to a room immediately. I took a seat in the room and Mum stood behind me. Uncle Richard entered the room, gave Mum a peck on the check and took a seat in his chair. As he sat, he directed a question to my mum as if I didn't exist. 'What's up with Sarah, Sue?' Mum answered on my behalf. He eventually asked me some close-ended questions to which I replied 'yes, no, maybe, sometimes, not really.' He wrote a prescription for amoxicillin, handed it to Mum and we left after they had finished their pleasantries.

We got into the car and Mum decided to stop by our family friends—David and Heather—who happened to own the local pharmacy. I waited in the car. I stared out the window again, the rain continuing to fall and hitting the glass on my side. I was transfixed by the falling rain and heard my father's words..

'You have all the answers inside of you. All you have to do is ask the question and trust your answer.'

I asked myself what I needed right now and the answer to my surprise came back with 'rest'.

Umm, I thought.

Mum returned to the car and we headed home. As soon as we were in the door Mum went straight to the kitchen cupboard, grabbed a glass, filled it with water, popped the tablet from the packet and slid both across the kitchen bench.

'There you go, darling, this will make you feel better.'

I looked Mum square in the eyes, much like my dad had done to me, with certainty and knowing and said 'No, thank you, I'm going to rest in my room,' and off I went.

After I said 'no' that eventful day, a new girl started at school and we became friends. We used to constantly stay at each other's house during the week. I loved going to her house; her mum seemed different to mine. Not better, just different.

Although her mother was a nurse and in the allopathic system she was open to different ways of looking at health compared to our family. There used to be bottles of 'things' in her fridge. I remember sitting at their kitchen bench, firing question after question to her mum wanting to know more about the bottles of things that rattled. Of course I thought they were tablets because of the sound, however I noted that the packaging was different. She shared with me that they were vitamins. 'Vitamins?' I asked. 'What are they?' She explained what vitamins were and how important they were for the body. I was mesmerised as I sat and listened intently to what she was sharing about the human body and health, all of which made sense to me and spurred on my interest in health.

 Ah ha!

- Map your life and note the pivotal changes—what doors opened and which ones closed?
- Who were the people, places, events or ideas that instigated a change in your thinking?

CHAPTER 4

Vital Moms Takes Flight...

'The pendulum of the mind alternates between sense
and nonsense, not between right and wrong.'

—— Carl Jung

March of 2010 ...

Randall was preparing dinner and I was buried in the fridge attempting to find the vegetable he'd requested. While searching the fridge I said to Randall, 'Something is going to happen in July. I can feel it. I'm not sure what it is but I know it's coming and it's going to change your life, my life, our children's lives and the lives of children around the world.'

I passed Randall the vegetables. 'Ooookay,' said Randall.

I didn't think much more of it either.

Over the following weeks I thought the energy I was feeling was tied to the events I was setting up at the time in the United Kingdom, United States, Australia and New Zealand teaching health professionals about running a vitalistic business. As July was fast approaching my mind was on establishing the layout of the events: content, additional speakers, location, invitations, tickets. My mind certainly wasn't on the conversation I'd had with Randall back in March.

I began noticing *every time* I wrote a deadline on my wall calendar the calendar would fall off the wall. I'd pick it up and stick it back to the wall. Down it would come again. This went on for two months.

I could feel the energy rise and a wave begin to swell. But I carried on with getting the events organised, thinking this was 'the thing' that was going to change the lives of children around the world.

Five days before my 43rd birthday …

I was sitting at home working and the kids were lying on the couch. They weren't at the nanny's house that day.

The nanny arrived at our place with some sugared lozenges, orange and propolis (a 'natural' antibiotic) for the children because she thought they were sick.

'Would you give these to the children?' she asked.

I read the ingredients.

'No,' I said, and told her why.

She left, went back to the chemist, brought some different lozenges—Manuka honey—and returned thirty minutes later asking if I would give them these other ones that were more expensive and apparently better quality.

I again read the ingredients and said 'No'.

'Why not?' she asked, espousing the healing benefits of Manuka Honey. I told her and we ended up having a brief discussion about squashing symptoms that the body created to alert a person to changes that are taking place. She wasn't happy with the discussion and brought up vaccinations. I sensed that she was not open to conversation nor willing at that point to look at health differently in that moment. I thanked her for her concern and she left.

I immediately rang Randall, concerned that she'd been at our place 'pushing an over-the-counter medication to take something away'.

'I have a feeling she'll ring CYFS (child youth and family services),' I said.

'She wouldn't do that,' said Randall.

I felt a little weird and attempted to lay to rest the thoughts swirling in my head.

Three days before my 43rd birthday …

Two days later Rui and Anais, our two youngest, were a little chirpier and they both said they would go to the nanny's. Anam, our eldest, who was still working through his health expression (sickness) said he would like to stay at home and sleep. Randall dropped the two little ones off and Anam promptly went back to sleep upstairs in our bed near my study space.

About 9:30 am, Anam was sound asleep and I was on the phone with two of my existing team members, interviewing a potential additional team member. As I sat in my pyjamas, listening and asking questions of the candidate, in walked our nanny with Rui and Anais. I thought Randall and I had forgotten to pack an item like a jumper or a rain jacket. I saw her march past the kitchen and into our bedroom. I immediately sensed that something was not right. I excused myself from the conversation, thought I muted the phone line (which I didn't) and called out 'Is everything okay?'

By the time I got to her, she had walked out of the bedroom to the kitchen, opened the freezer door, taken Anam's fish bait, walked back to the bedroom and placed the frozen bait on his forehead. I knew there was something not right going on and hung up on the phone call, not to return to it.

I stood in the middle of the passageway watching this take place. I walked into our bedroom where she was standing and Anam was lying. I noticed she'd pulled the bed covers off him, waking him up. She said,'I can't believe he has bed covers on him, winter pyjamas and hot water bottles in bed with him; he's as hot as anything.'

My son looked at me with puzzled eyes having never, at the age of eight, had anyone place anything on his forehead. My gaze back was reassuring: *I'm here; you're safe.* I mentioned to her it's winter, he is in my bed and the water bottles were now cold having been in there the night before. I followed her back to the lounge room and stood, frozen, wondering what was going to happen next as she paced the floor.

She turned on me again, bullying me, standing in my space and right in my face and pointed at Rui who was five years old and crouched behind the couch protecting his three-year-old sister while peeking around the corner, staring at me with terrified eyes. I glanced back in the same way I did with our eldest, reassuring him and his sister: *I'm here; you're safe.*

'Do you know he has a *temperature*?' said the nanny, pointing at Rui. 'And?'

'His temperature is 38.7°C.' (101.66)

'And?'

'Well, that is dangerously high and he could have a fit.'

'According to who?' I said.

She continued talking. I went numb, transported out of my body to a 10,000-foot view where I could see the event taking place in a world of quiet. Her voice became slightly muffled and I could only hear my voice saying, 'It's July. This is the moment. This is the event that has been organising around you to change your life and the lives of individuals, families and children around the world.'

As soon as I stopped hearing my own voice and seeing the big view, I was immediately transported back to my body and returned to hearing hers ...

'I have no choice but to call CYFS.'

As I stood in front of her I realized this was it. This was the event—not the live events around the world I was coordinating. This was THE live event that would change my life, my family's life and the lives of children around the world. 'Don't do that,' I said. Part of me wanted to roar, but inside I felt so much shock that she would even say that. I believed it was something we could sort out.

In a blink my life changed.

As soon as she left, the kids ran to me and I formed a huge protective shield with my arms around them all. The tears began to pour out, a symphony of uncontrollable crying as we attempted to make sense of what just took place. The events swirled in our heads with not a word spoken. I slowly pulled myself together and called my husband.

I continued to hold them close as I rang Randall, barely able to breathe, crying through the phone. Randall could hear our little girl howling in the background and all I could stutter, gasping for breath was the name of our nanny and CYFS. My husband's rage was palpable through the phone. He screamed, 'Tell her to *get the fuck out of our house.*'

Randall apologised to the practice members sitting in the reception area, saying 'My family needs me. I have to go. Would you mind rescheduling?'

They, of course, all said yes. Before he left CYFS had called the practice; I hadn't answered the phone at home and the nanny must have given them both numbers.

Moments later he walked through the front door. My vacant stare must have said it all. Randall didn't say anything; he simply gathered us together in his arms and, rocking us back and forth, he said over and over, 'I love you all, you're safe now. I love you all, you're safe now.' I was numb, catatonic, as I sat tucked into his arms, my eyes red from crying and speechless.

The nanny had been in our employ for two years; her employment ceased that day.

She knew our approach to health: no drugs, no medications (prescription or over-the-counter) and no medical intervention. No 'this for that'. Our children have been taught since birth that the power that made the body heals the body. They have also been taught to embrace whatever they've created for themselves as an opportunity to grow.

At 1:00 pm on July 22nd the phone call came through.

When my tears had settled slightly my husband informed me that CYFS have placed us on a 'critical list' because we were 'denying children the right to medical treatment'. Randall had informed CYFS that as doctors of chiropractic we serve vast numbers of children including our own, and as such we know when our children have temperatures and when they don't and in this particular instance they DO NOT have temperatures, and perhaps the nanny got it wrong.

CYFS were adamant in telling us that our only option to clear our name off the 'critical list' was to take our children to a medical doctor to verify that they in fact did not have temperatures. All of a sudden our right to choose what health approach we wanted for ourselves and our children was being threatened. We were being told what to do.

I rang friends across the world to locate medical doctors who would assist us and support us in our choices. As I was calling, my husband had made a call to the local medical practice on the island where we live, the same medical practice that had used our services in the past to educate their community on health. The medical practice co-ordinator was lovely, very obliging and sensitive to our situation. She was familiar with our views on health and where it comes from and asked one of the medical doctors more aligned to our way of thinking to open her books up so she could see us. This medical doctor said yes and, like us, wanted to get it taken care of that day so the family could move on.

By 3:00 pm we were at the medical doctor's and I was out to quietly prove a point … *that our children DID NOT have temperatures.* Before we went to the medical doctor's I sat my children on the couch and said, 'Kids, we're about to jump through some hoops. Today will be a new experience for us all and it will no doubt bring up lots of questions for us as a family to answer together. Today is your first appointment with a medical doctor and she will be jumping through the hoop with us.'

So off we went as a family, ready to have an experience.

When we arrived, Robyn, the practice coordinator was very kind and took us immediately to their administration room saying, 'You don't have to wait out there. This will be a lot more comfortable for you. I'll come and get you when the doctor is ready.'

Eventually it was our turn. Robyn showed us through to the doctor's room. She spoke to the kids a little, took their temperatures and, no surprise to us, the temperatures were normal … 36.8°C (98.24°F), 37.2°C (98.96°F) and 38°C (100.4°F). The doctor rang CYFS to give them the temperatures of the children.

We breathed again. It was all over … *or so we thought.*

Little did we know that when you enter CYFS you lose some of your rights over your children. You are left in the lurch. No one contacts you, no one lets you know when your 'status' has changed. CYFS told us that if we took our children to a medical doctor to get their temperature checked they would take us off the critical list.

Days went by. No one called or returned our calls to let us know if our names had been cleared from the 'critical list' so we could get on with life.

Eventually, through our own persistence we got in contact with the young CYFS lady who initially called us. She said, 'Yes, this appears to be an unsubstantiated allegation and we're going to close your case.' Randall said thank you and hung up.

I was at the practice when the phone rang, and I could barely understand the high pitched, stuttering, shallow breathing voice on the end of the phone *they called and they have closed the allegation*. I asked twice 'who is this?'. Eventually I understood who it was and heard the words again *they called and they have closed the allegation*. I cried with my husband. Through my tears I said, 'Let's celebrate tonight with the kids. I'll be home shortly.'

When I arrived home Randall and I sat on the couch and called the kids into the lounge room. We told them the allegation against us was now closed. The kids one at a time moved towards us, my husband gathering them up with his outstretched arms. Holding each other tightly we shed our tears in silence; a feeling of relief flooded us all. We decided to take the kids out for their favourite meal— Indian—and we picked up a movie on the way home. Ironically the movie they chose was 'Nanny McPhee'.

Our kids didn't want to be further than earshot from us nor separated from each other. So we kept their sleeping arrangements as it had been since the CYFS call came through—mattresses snuggled together in the adjoining room to ours, camping on the floor. We went to bed, relieved and exhausted; the kids were all together. We wanted it that way too. We all slept soundly thinking life can step forward now.

We awoke from the best sleep we had all had in two weeks. Just after breakfast the phone rang. It was CYFS informing us there had been a mistake, a misunderstanding at their end, that in fact the allegation was NOT closed. They informed us they would be coming over to the island to meet with us.

Suddenly the requirements and the rules had changed; allegation open, allegation closed, allegation re-opened *and now they were coming to our house.*

They then told us it wasn't one person coming across, it was two.

'What for?' I screamed at my husband. 'Why are they coming here and why are they changing the rules?' I felt like a lion roaring to protect the cubs. Randall wasn't sure. In his mind he was attempting to make sense of it all too. We spoke to CYFS, telling them we had no other option but to protect our children and ourselves and that we would now be seeking legal counsel.

After dialing a few people to locate a lawyer who would support us in our views and circumstances they all said, 'You don't want a lawyer; get a friend to come over and scribe the meeting, telling them that they can get a copy.' The following week when they arrived at our house we introduced our 'friend'.

They told us this was a 'routine visit' and when they go back to their offices this afternoon the case would be more than likely closed given the unsubstantiated allegation against us. Before that could happen, however, the two young ladies had to have a meeting with their supervisor and other colleagues to approve the closure, which they said would happen that afternoon.

It took another seven weeks for CYFS to return our calls and close the case.

No one knew what was happening. The lady who was overseeing our case had gone on holiday and no one had taken the time to call us, return our calls or let us know the case was closed. This resulted in a huge amount of emotional stress for ourselves, our kids, as a married couple and as parents ... the not knowing despite them saying it was an unsubstantiated allegation.

When I spoke to the lady at CYFS I was calm but clear: *this was absolutely an unsubstantiated allegation against us and the manner in which it had been handled was even worse.* I stayed calm because I knew I had only just begun sharing this story.

During the three months I felt I was 'fighting' CYFS I felt this momentous urge *to organise the world's health information into bite-sized pieces so people can understand it.* Clearly the nanny and us had a different understanding of health and I wanted to know on what basis people made their health decisions. I attempted to find a system of understanding within the question of 'how do people approach health?' The information began to flood my mind as I became more and more open to be the vessel for the knowledge; now I just had to organise it so people could understand it.

During the time it took for CYFS to close the case I disappeared; off the radar. I rarely ventured in to our small community on the island, stepped immediately out of practice and spent every day with our kids. Every time I drove past the nanny my stomach sank, anger would percolate and I'd wondered if she knew the kids DIDN'T have temperatures the eventful day she called CYFS. An additional allegation she made had to do with home educating our children. When it came to education, like health, she had a different understanding and approach. Pure and simply, I ran. I felt lied to and cheated and extremely scared and paranoid about what people in a small community would be saying. I didn't want to be the one to kill our bricks and mortar business we were growing so I decided to hone my energies on the USA clients I had so as to be as far away from the people in my own backyard. I blocked them out. I thought everyone I was meeting in our community knew of our situation. I was paranoid. And that is the main reason why 'Vital Moms' is spelt with an 'O' rather than a 'U' even though both spellings will get you to the website.

With the 'case' now closed I was ready to let everyone know about the three different approaches to health and how to gain trust and feel confident in making the right health decisions. During the three months it took to close the case I wrote over 60,000 words, all of which contributed to forming Vital Moms. I am proud to say that my 'event' and the knowledge I was open to receiving during this time has now assisted thousands upon thousands of individuals and families in over 32 countries to approach health differently and to gain confidence with the decisions they make. You, as a responsible parent and individual, have the right to choose what health approach you want to use for either yourself or your child.

Since my 'event' I've dedicated my time to educating individuals and parents about the different approaches to health and what health truly is. And there's nothing like an event that you had a hand in creating that enlarges your purpose.

 Ah ha!

* Name a significant event you created in your life that shook you to the core but sparked action in an unforeseen direction and as a result now sees you helping people?

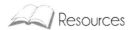 Resources

'Fevers: don't use Paracetamol'
www.VitalMoms.com/healthillusion

CHAPTER 5

Confronting the Nanny

*'In any area of your life where you feel
disempowered someone will overpower you.'*

—— Dr John Demartini

Tuesday 27th August, 2013 @ 5:25 pm

For the past three months I'd wanted to speak with the nanny who had called CYFS. I didn't know when it would be, I just felt it was coming; it was time. I felt that I should speak with her to close the situation; to stop feeling the anger, trepidation and the horrid thought of bumping into her in the small community I lived in.

It wasn't too long beforehand that my husband and I had helped our two boys stand up to bullies within their circle of friends, giving them the skills, a new angle to view their situation and a conversation 'structure' to assist them with what *they* wanted to do.

I'm grateful to our kids and their bullies because it stirred in me my own incongruence. Since those conversations with the boys the nanny and the CYFS situation began percolating to the surface.

My internal chatter became clearer and clearer 'Speak to her, close it once and for all; for yourself.'

There were a few times I could have approached her—car parks, street, market—however every time I looked at her I was torn by the overwhelming need to approach her and the feeling of a mild earthquake inside: blood pressure increasing, heart beat racing and sudden sweating. I knew I wasn't ready for such an encounter. So I waited and became the observer of my emotions. I noticed more and more that each time I saw her my emotional response lessened.

And then the day arrived ...

I dropped Anam at dance; he was about to begin a new genre of dance with the group he performs with. I thought I would stay and watch it to get a feel for what he would be learning. The nanny had arrived to drop another child off. I sat watching the new dance genre while chatting to one of the mums. Time flew by and before I knew it, the nanny was there again. An overwhelming feeling of *it's now or never* came over me. I checked in with my body and observed that there was no fast heart beat, no sweating, no mini earthquake occurring. I was ready.

The nanny left and headed for her car. I called her name and she turned around.

'I know we haven't spoken in quite some time but I wanted to say "Thank you" for what you did.'

'Why are you thanking me?'

'Because I had the opportunity to educate people at CYFS about health and I have been able to now build a global business that helps lots of mothers and families look at health differently.'

'Well, that is a bit pathetic, thanking me. Why are you doing that?'

'Because I am grateful you made that phone call.'

'Well I would do it again'.

'That is neither here nor there for me, I just want to thank you.'

'Basically I did it out of fear because your child had a temperature and you're a neglectful parent.'

'The children actually didn't have temperatures.'

'Yes he did. I took his temperature and it was very high and he was sweating.'

'We took them to a medical doctor to have their temperatures taken immediately upon receiving the CYFS call. The temperatures of all three were normal.

'Well that is ridiculous.'

'The medical doctor said ALL were normal. I was there and I've received a copy of what they wrote down.'

'I'm a trained pediatric nurse, I know how to take temperatures. Anyway you do all that alternative health which is so unscientific.'

'That is your opinion. All I wanted to say was thank you.'

'Well, you don't have to.'

'For me, I do.'

She got in her car. As I got into my car I was shaking like a leaf. I settled my body down before driving, and chatted with Anais immediately so she could process what portion of the conversation she heard. Many people may feel that it was not appropriate for a child to bear witness to a conversation such as this. However there were valuable lessons and being a family that places all conversations and emotions on the table to be spoken about enabled us all to feel complete. I felt free at last to be within the community I have chosen to be part of. Part of me was shaking and in shock that I had actually done it, however also proud of myself for having done so.

When I got home I sat on my chair in my study, hugged Rui and Anais and shared what had taken place. We smiled and cried at the same time. When I returned to dance about thirty minutes later to collect Anam, I shared with him about what I had done. He simply said, 'I am proud of you Mum.'

I posted this message on my Vital Moms facebook page:

I just did something that has taken me three years to do. I approached the nanny that called CYFS (child services) on us. I did so with trepidation, apprehension and fear—I did it anyway. Not long ago I taught our child to stand up to those who bully. I felt incongruent with what I was saying and doing, wondering why it has taken me three years to do so. TODAY was the day. Although I am grateful I had the full gamut of emotions sweeping through me, NOW I feel liberated like the rape person who heads to jail to thank the perpetrator. I am grateful that this experience had me develop Vital Moms, a place for parents and individuals who are wanting to approach health differently. A place for those who feel like the lone parent or person with a community against what they believe, or worse yet, a family against them. I wanted to give the people a voice, a place to learn, empowering themselves with a greater understanding of health, the human body and its expression. And above all feel supported in the decisions they make. I'm grateful ... I now feel complete.

 Ah ha!

* Live congruently with your thoughts and actions.
* Take the time to see where situations in your life need 'clearing up', to set you free to be the person you were destined to be.

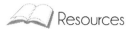 Resources

'The bully or the bullied'
www.VitalMoms.com/healthillusion

CHAPTER 6

Medical Obedience?

'We have learned all the answers, all the answers:
it is the questions that we do not know.'
—— Archibald MacLeish

When my blinkers were on I thought health was about how you
felt … period. If your body looked and felt taut, tight and terrific and
no signs or symptoms were present then, according to my world and
the books I read, you were 'healthy'. How naïve I was back then. I was
led to believe for the first ten years of my life that health was given
to me by something and/or someone other than myself. Indeed,
health was given to me from the outside-in by things I consumed
(medications) or things I did (physical fitness, eating good food,
positive thoughts and being in a happy state) all of which determined
my level and expression of health … or so I thought. There was a
simple unspoken rule—a 'medical obedience'—that governed my
life and the lives of those around me. It was this: 'if you're sick, take
something … it will make you better.'

When 'it' (symptom/s) wasn't there anymore I was deemed by myself, my parents, peers and the private school I attended to be healthy once again.

In fact, I thought health existed on a spectrum.

The Oxford Dictionary defines Spectrum as follows:

'A spectrum is used to classify something in terms of

its position on a scale between two extreme points.'

This positional interpretation of health made sense, given the unspoken medical obedience rule I lived by: 'if you're sick, take something... it will make you better,' thereby keeping you nudged towards the right end; the top end where 'health' sits. So for the first ten years of my life **I obeyed this unspoken medical obedience rule without question** and did whatever I could to stay at the top end of the health spectrum which meant consuming medication after medication to make me 'feel' better.

The health spectrum I obeyed looked like this:

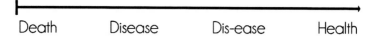

Death   Disease   Dis-ease   Health

Interestingly, at the tender age of seven I was told by my father that I had all the answers inside of me. All I had to do was ask the question and trust my answer. These were two very conflicting ways of not only looking at my health, but my life as well. On the one hand the actions and observations of my family taught me that I was incomplete and incapable of changing my own health and as a result I was offered, and consumed various medications to take whatever 'it' was away. And on the other hand I was told I had all the answers; all I had to do was ask a question and trust my answer. This implied that indeed I was capable of knowing why something had been created within me and that I could change my circumstance if I wanted to.

At the age of ten, I'd experienced that incident where I coughed a couple of times, was whisked off to my uncle's medical practice, and given a prescription for amoxicillin. For the first time in my short life I refused to take a medication my mum had offered me. Little did I know that asking the question and trusting my answer that eventful day, 'saying no' to my mum and going to my bedroom to rest, would change the course of my life.

Most importantly as I got older I wanted to know how people were defining health, what drives people to make the health decisions they do, how does the body express health and who really is molding the way society sees health? It wasn't until I began studying Psychology and eventually Chiropractic that my encounters with some extraordinary professors, people and authors began to open different worlds for me.

Shortly after the home birth of our second child, Rui, I was, as a health professional, witnessing more and more parents pressured to 'toe the line' with medical obedience and medicate their children. These parents were being told by professionals within the allopathic community—doctors and nurses—that they were irresponsible parents if they didn't do 'X', 'Y' and 'Z'; perpetuating 'what if' scenarios and fear in their minds. As a result of hearing this time and time again, I made it my mission to find out how people were defining health.

I buckled Rui my newborn and Anam my than toddler into the car, packed up the pram and some refreshments, nappies, water bottle, a clipboard and pen and drove to our local shopping centre. Upon arriving, I piled up the pram and headed for the busiest corner I knew of in the shopping centre. I popped Rui in the baby sling and, with Anam close by, stopped anybody walking past who looked at me.

I asked one simple question: 'What is health?'

After quite a few hours of stopping and chatting with people I packed up and drove home. I immediately went and placed all the responses on my desk and didn't think much more of it until later that evening when the kids were asleep. The responses were interesting. I was looking for a pattern, a system; something that I could extrapolate from the experience and use to educate people on the way in which most people see health.

I separated all the responses, grouping each according to common themes. I found there were five top responses which I concluded was society's definition of health. They all certainly had an element of the 'unspoken rule' I was raised with ... how we define health says a great deal about how we approach it.

The top five responses were:

1) Health is having no signs or symptoms.

2) Health is having no pain.

3) Health is about eating well.

4) Health is about being fit and exercising.

5) Health is about being happy.

All of these responses confirm the belief of health existing on a *spectrum* and the preference for one to stay towards the 'right' end of it. In other words you don't want to experience the opposite of any of those top five responses.

It was in a philosophy class in the 1990s while studying at Palmer that the 'health spectrum' bubble *exploded* for me. In this philosophy class my teacher had shared a different definition of health. I had not come across this definition before simply because of how I was choosing to see health; however it was there all along. It was from Dorland's Medical Dictionary and it also happens to be the definition adopted by the Chiropractic profession and by the World Health Organisation. It says health is …

> 'Optimum physical, mental and social wellbeing and not necessarily the absence of disease and infirmity.'
> — *Dorland's Pocket Medical Dictionary*

Would you agree that these are two vastly different ways to look at health?

On the one hand you are seen as a machine and the approach to your health is very mechanistic, confined to medical obedience … 'Here, take this. It will make you feel better.' You are viewed as a person with many parts, and as such medications are given to deal with the parts, e.g. constipation means laxatives, headaches means vasodilators (e.g. Panadol), eczema means cortisone creams, asthma means puffers filled with ephedrine or epinephrine. And so forth. You are offered anything to keep you tipped towards the 'right end'.

Let's take a brief look inside the human body to acknowledge an often overlooked vital perspective on health that is consistently left out of health literature. This vital perspective acknowledges that within the human body there are concurrently both good and bad 'things' occurring. For instance, there are toxic (negative) and tonic (positive) reactions occurring within the body at the exact same time. There are also chemical changes across cell membranes: one could be deemed good because of the positive charge—Sodium, $Na+$—and the other one deemed bad because of the negative charge—Potassium, K^-. There is also cell growth, labeled as good because it refers to growth, and cell death, bad because it refers to death. All are occurring in the body at the *exact same time*.

So does health exist as a spectrum or on a continuum?

The truth is … health exists on a continuum. Your body exists with BOTH health and disease. In fact you cannot have one without the other just like there is no high tide without a low tide, sunrise without a sunset, males without females and light without dark. The root meaning of the word 'health' means 'wholeness'. In other words, to be whole there must be two sides—a positive (good) and a negative (bad)—that when joined make the complete whole. When we acknowledge this truth we acknowledge that the body does not know health until it knows disease and vice versa. Inherent within this is the health continuum.

'Continuum' as defined by the Merriam Webster Dictionary is:

'a range or series of things that are slightly different from each other and that exist between two different possibilities.'

And in Latin *Continuum* from the 1600s means 'a continuous thing' and *Continue* from the 1300s literally means 'to hang together'.

Umm … interesting.

By chasing the pain free, symptom free, disease free approach to health you shall, by the very virtue of your actions, diminish your health. The health continuum, as I call it, is the acknowledgement that we aren't just sick or well but that our health is continuously *changing and oscillating* along a continuum that expresses all aspects of health (wholeness) all the time, day in and day, out for the whole of our physical existence. So at times we might be at either end or somewhere in between. The fluctuations in our health expression create our own unique and personal health continuum. There is NO one cookie cutter health continuum. Our personal and unique health expression is an experience expressed via our own personal perceptions of our seven areas of life: spiritual, mental, vocational, familial, financial, social and physical. The emphasis is on *oscillate* and most of the time we aren't even aware of the movement and changes that take place; our remarkable innate (inborn) intelligence, which runs our body, is simply taking care of it. There comes a time, however, when our innate intelligence gives our educated mind the awareness of how we are living and this is when symptoms become known to us at a conscious level. Factors within the body, as well as our perceptual understanding of our environment, are seen to be the most important in bringing about change along the continuum in either direction.

When working with people I look inside to find factors that are preventing adaptation to the outside world. I acknowledge that a person is more able to adapt by being present to the environment than by avoiding it. Remember the definition of health (wholeness) says ... *'and not necessarily the absence of disease of infirmity.'*

 Ah ha!

* Name five ways you are living a life of 'medical obedience'?

CHAPTER 7

Do You Have the Nerve to be Healthy?

'Anything's possible if you've got enough nerve.'
— JK Rowling

Before you discover if you have the nerve to be healthy you have to first ask the question, 'What is health?' Most people across a variety of professions interpret health as how we feel, what we eat, what we look like, and whether we can run around the block. I know because I was in this sector of the 'health industry' for decades. I even did a year and a half of enrolled study at Deakin University in Victoria, Australia studying to be a dietician. I swiftly realised that wasn't for me when I'd driven down to Geelong (Deakin Campus) for the day to attend a class workshop. In this workshop we were discussing 'fats' and we had to go around two tables individually and rate the various fat items on display according to their nutritional value and 'health goodness'. In one session on 'spreadable butters' my fellow students and I, with clipboards in hand, had to rate butter and a plethora of margarine brands as to which was better for health according to the ingredients. Most chose margarine which at the time, according to the food pyramid, great marketing, dietitians, nutritionists, big Pharma and a plethora of other 'health' professionals was the correct answer. I however chose butter ... which was, according to them, wrong. I was given a 'talking to' and no matter how much I defended my stance, it simply fell on deaf ears. I sat the exam that was fast approaching after this one day workshop, and failed. I answered the questions according to what common, logical sense would deem plausible, choosing answers that came from nature rather than from a laboratory, knowing that if you eat enough of the food made by the people in the white coats you'll end up seeing the people in the white coats. I hop footed it out of Deakin and never looked back.

I was still, however, caught in my bubble of health being about how someone felt and would constantly ask clients at the gym I worked at how they felt! I remember one gentleman, Tony, who used to come to my early morning circuit classes and he couldn't for the life of him stretch his hamstrings. I kept telling him 'Tony it's not good for your body, you need to be able to stretch!' I gave him a whole lot of exercises to work on, nutritional advice and emotional support for the issues he was going through.

However, one thing I couldn't do back then was tell him what health was. Why? Because I had never been taught it.

Well actually that's not entirely true.

I had been taught health via my parent's actions. The actions which my parents demonstrated when someone was 'sick' and the observations I made about those actions taught me what health was. I learnt from a young age that health is about how you feel—you go to someone (more educated than you) to get something (medications) to take something away (signs and symptoms) to make you healthy (feeling good) and that this lineal domino process is not questioned. Everyone does it and therefore so will we. No questions asked.

Inherent in this teaching method are incongruences that cross over into other parenting paths. For instance if your child comes to you and says 'Everybody else is doing x, y and z; why can't I?' your initial response, I imagine, will be 'Because as your parents we are choosing to do a, b and c instead.' Your response demonstrates that something outside of the family is not going to dictate what goes on in the family, nor are you going to have your children blindly follow other people. However ... when it comes to health we blindly follow, without question, doing what all the other people do. Following the herd equals a life of mediocrity, and mediocre health too.

There was an underlying suggestion that when you studied physical education and/or were associated with sport in some way that you simply knew what it was—feelings, food and fitness. But, I never once stopped to ask myself 'what innervates our muscles ... what switches them on?' until I went to Palmer, where one of my first health illusions to be broken was my persistent misunderstood definition of health: feelings, food and fitness.

I also learnt:

> 1) that we are self-healing, self-regulating organisms that are constantly adapting to our environment. When we are unable to adapt to the life around us we create changes in our physiology which in turn create the signs and symptoms that we experience. Mind blowing moment!

and;

> 2) the nerve system is the master communicating system of the body; it is what we use to sense our world and adapt and it's the one that coordinates all our functions.

You can imagine how this floored me. Never before had I heard health defined in terms of optimum possibility and function. My jaw dropped, my eyes boggled and I felt like a kangaroo in headlights—stunned! When I left the philosophy class I threw my old definition of health—feelings, food and fitness—out the window. I walked around college floating on cloud nine solidly connected to my percolating belief in the body's incredible power to express health *with and without disease*. Although I had stopped attending medical doctors decades prior to entering Palmer, I found I was still allowing my old way of interpreting health—feelings, food and fitness—to govern my views. As a result I found it a challenge to live congruently with my new understanding. I knew at the time it was imperative to make additional 'shifts' in my thinking.

I had another illusion of mine broken fairly swiftly. It was made very clear to me that *all* the functions of the body only worked to the ability of the electrical supply (nerve system, the master communicating system). In other words, any given system of the body is only as strong as its weakest link. We were taught the nerve system is the electrical supply (the wires), and there is not one thing you can do in your body without neurological innervation. I understood that the nerve system was *the over arching key* in a series of intricate and well-designed individual nerves (wires) leading in many different directions. There are thousands and thousands of nerves, all of which come together at the base of the skull to form the spinal cord. These nerves go to every cell, tissue, organ and system of the body. There is 100% co-ordinated activity and communication between them all and your expression of health is proportionate to the function of your nerve supply. So where does health come from? The inside, of course.

When you take a closer look at the nerve system—the body's communication system —you'll notice a series of intricate and well-designed wires leading in many different directions. To the untrained eye it would seem chaotic, but to the trained eye it is one of the most remarkable systems you could ever have the pleasure of viewing. While studying, I was able to fuel my obsession with the human body during our cadaver classes which we had for approximately two years. I also taught other students in the cadaver lab for two and a half of the years which reinforced for me the intricacies of the nerve system. I used to drift off at times and visualise that the person lying there was alive and I was able to 'see' one of their tiny cells and the twelve different nerve fibres innervating it with an average of 100,000 synaptic endings for every nerve fibre making over 1.2 million nerve endings that were constantly hooking up in various intricate ways to innervate one cell! I'd soon 'snap' back to it after intellectually stimulating my visual cortex and wondering what life would be like as a nerve impulse racing over the fibers. The body knows what to do every time, one hundred percent of the time, provided there is no interference to our key system—the nerve system. (See Chapter 9: The Health Illusion)

Have you ever noticed a sun rise and a sun set; a high tide and a low tide; summer and winter; light and dark? Sure you have. And what did you notice? Did you notice you can't have one without the other? Internally, inside of ourselves, you also have a balanced world. You have in your body an opportunity for feedback. This closed circuit is in constant communication with your innate intelligence, your educated mind and your nerve system. It's called homeostasis. Homeostasis enables you to adapt to your environment internally and externally. The balance inherent within your internal world is demonstrated by your cells growing and dying at the same time; toxic and tonic reactions occurring at the same time and ever-so-minute amounts of positive and negative charged particles crossing cell membranes in absolute perfect balance, so as to keep the extracellular and the intracellular fluids in balance.

Let's look at health from this functional definition of optimum opportunity and potential (Dorland's definition) and the question to ask is 'Can you gain health by getting rid of disease?'

The answer is 'No!'

Why? Well disease, just like the functional definition says, is necessary for the optimum expression of your health. You require it in order to grow and adapt to your life. What would life be like if we had no disease? What would life be like if there was no darkness, just sunlight? You have both sides in your life, in your body and there's a reason for them. Dis-ease and disease are created by yourself as a gift to nudge you in a different direction, open different doors and assist with an opportunity to adapt and evolve in your life. Don't be afraid to make the change because of what you perceive you will lose … because you will also gain.

Let's look at it this way:

If I handed you a magnet and said 'Chop off the negative end,' could you do it?

The answer is 'No!' you can't.

Why? Because they exist together and when you look closely you see that within the negative is the positive and within the positive is the negative; they co-exist. In an allopathic world the body is only equal to the sum of its parts, believing that the smallest component of matter is the atom which has no intelligence or consciousness. Coinciding with this interpretation of the human body is this understanding that all 'things' inside of you are independent from one another; that indeed there is no overarching system that governs their function. It assumes, too, that everybody is the same on the inside which, of course, is not true.

Your level of function is determined by how you respond to your unique thoughts (i.e. emotions: perceptions, beliefs and interpretation of life), your trauma experiences (i.e. physical: birth, falls, accidents), and toxins (i.e. chemicals: food, air, smoke, household chemicals). You truly are as different on the inside as you are on the outside.

Do you have the nerve to be healthy?

 Ah ha!

* Are you ready to see how your body expresses health with and without disease?

* Look at the different ways your level of function may be determined by the unique combination of thoughts, trauma and toxins.

CHAPTER 8

What is Your Family Health Recipe?

'The shoe that fits one person pinches another; there is no recipe for living that suits all cases.'

—— Carl Jung

It is time to lift the veil on the way health has always been interpreted and provide a new way to view health that paints a truthful and incredible picture of the human potential and possibility. This will, in turn, give you renewed confidence in your body's ability to express health according to you and arm you with options.

Many people don't stop to question health, following the old saying of 'if it works why change it?' or 'if it ain't broke, don't fix it.' The health challenge to come for future generations is to clearly understand what health is and the capabilities and possibilities of the human body, including the mind.

The current, most accepted and utilised approach to health merely masks that which the body wants us to acknowledge and change.

Even our car has warning lights to alert us to take action. The orange petrol (gas) warning light pops up when we are low on petrol, you hear a 'beeping' sound when a door is left open and a small genie type bottle appears on the dashboard when the oil needs a top up; all there to indicate that YOU must take action and do something in order to change the current circumstances of your car. Or you can stop on the side of the road, pull out some masking tape you may have in your glove box and place a strip of masking tape across the dash board, cut the wires so you no longer hear the 'beep' sound, hope for the best and 'soldier on' as they say until you completely ruin the engine. At this stage you then blame everyone and everything else including the masking tape YOU chose to place on the dashboard and the scissors you used to cut the wire, all because you weren't willing to take responsibility and make the changes required.

Your body is a lot more intricate than a car engine.

Over eighty-five per cent of the health challenges diagnosed in society today are generated by lifestyle. That means you have the innate power within you to change it simply by looking closely at how you live and the choices you are making. However, more and more people are being diagnosed with diabetes, Alzheimer's, heart disease, arthritis, depression, stroke, high cholesterol, high blood pressure, metabolic syndrome, asthma, eczema, irritable bowel, gluten intolerance and more.

Why?

Well, there are many reasons as to why a person is unable or unwilling to change, including not knowing where to start (see beginning 'How to use this book to get the most out of it'). I believe there is unequivocally one place where you must start: it is your belief about what health is and where it comes from. In order to understand your approach to health I'm going to use an analogy of 'the family recipe,' but let me define it first.

Your family health recipe is …

'the subliminal messages (hidden messages acting on your subconscious) that took place in your life via a mother, father, teacher, preacher, caregiver, TV, radio, print and now social media that sees you approaching health in the same way it was subliminally taught to you … without question … because that's the way it was always done.'

Here's a scenario to make the point. Let's say your family loves to bake.

Your grandmother is *the* best at making banana cake. Your grandmother was taught by her mother (your great-grandmother) who was taught by her mother (your great-great-grandmother); throughout the decades the recipe hasn't changed. It has been adhered to like a religion—*done that way because that's the way it's always been done.* As a young girl you stand by your mother in the kitchen, watching intently, observing her actions and listening closely to what she says as she mixes together the ingredients to bring the family banana cake to life. Eventually you grow, marry and have children of your own, at which time you start sharing the family recipe for banana cake—no notes, nothing written, barely anything said, shared with your daughter via your actions and the observations she makes of what you are doing. The art of unspoken learning and subliminal messages; done that way because that's the way it has always been done.

You were taught health in the same way.

You were taught via the actions of your parents when you were 'sick', the observations you made about their actions and you listened closely to the words, they used to describe what was happening when you were 'sick'. Essentially you grew up in a household that did health a certain way *without question* because that was the way it was always done; an insidious process in which people were not stopping to question.

To help it percolate some more, I'll say it again: the way you approach health now is more than likely the same way it was taught to you by your mother, father, teacher, preacher, caregiver, TV, radio, print media and now social media ... followed diligently, without question because that is the way it has always been done, unless you are stopping to question what you are doing and why.

Let me give you a simple and common example of learnt actions and observations.

I am sure if you have children you've done the internal 'Ouch!' as you've seen your child skidding off a bike. All children create opportunities for cuts and abrasions; whether it's falling off a bike, a scooter, a rock, from a tree, a skateboard or a surfboard. How you approach health and handle the situation, *the cut and the blood*, makes all the difference to what they will learn and believe about their own body and teach their own children when they come along. Remember the saying 'done that way because that's the way it has always been done'.

I remember as a young girl falling out of trees, grazing my knees, cutting the corner of my eye on the corner of a brick, jamming my finger in the car door and many other notable spills, trips and falls. I remember one vivid incident when I was quite young. I had been given a wonderful, brand new bike for Christmas—bright yellow, it was my favourite colour. I went riding to my friend's house a couple of blocks away to show it off to her. On my way home I attempted some new tricks, hit the road gutter, came off second best, fell and cut my knee. I walked home, crying all the way. I hobbled up the driveway, blood pouring from my knee, put my new bike near the back door and into the house I went bellowing 'Mummy, I'm bleeding.'

Mum, drawing on her 'family health recipe,' did the following:

She hugged me and told me I would be all right in an attempt to calm me down. She then picked me up and carried me to the bathroom to sit me on the side of the bath tub *(taught me that someone will take care of me)*. While I sat on the edge of the bath tub she grabbed some cotton wool from the medicine cabinet in the bathroom, wet it and with blood oozing from my knee said 'oh yucky' and proceed to wipe away the blood. 'There ... all clean now' she would say *(taught me that blood was not good and you have to stop it)*.

Mum would than take the Mercurochrome from the medicine cabinet, place a little on a cotton wool ball and dab it on my cut, staining my knee red. She would then get a sticky plaster (a.k.a. Band-Aid) to place on my knee. While opening the plaster wrapper she'd confidently say 'There you go, darling, this will make you feel better' as she stuck the plaster on my knee *(taught me that something other than myself would do the healing for me; surrendered responsibility to a sticky plaster much like the masking tape and the car dashboard. Ignored.)*

I'd smile back, hug her again and off we would go as if nothing had happened. What was communicated to me about health during these times could have had me stay firmly planted in the allopathic approach to health—outside-in—had it not been for my dad taking the time to teach me something different at the age of seven.

I've taught myself to interpret health from a different, vital health perspective and so the above scenario in our house looks like this:

Firstly, I hug our children, like my mum did and ask what happened. Like any child, when they see blood it creates a hyper response, usually in the form of loud crying. And it doesn't matter if the cut is minuscule or a larger one, any sight of blood seems to elicit the same response. I too, while hugging and allowing the blood to flow from the cut area, give them the space to tell me what happened.

After the story we observe together the site of the cut and the blood and by this time the energy has somewhat dissipated.

I then remind them about why the body bleeds after a cut ...

Whenever there is a cut the innate wisdom of the body will respond in the same way, with blood seeping, oozing or flowing out. The blood is required as part of the natural healing process. The blood flows naturally to remove from the site debris, dirt and grit. The size of the cut and its depth determines the amount of blood that will flow from the area. As the blood is allowed to flow, a whole cascade of *internal events* takes place to initiate platelet coagulation. 'What's that?' I hear you say ... well, this is where the blood begins to clump together and ever so slightly harden, closing the 'gap' where the cut is. This forms the first part of the scab. How long does this usually take? *Two minutes!* The same length of time it takes to place a cloth over the site and apply pressure, the difference is with a cloth the blood is not freely flowing which allows the body to innately remove the debris. The blood innately stops flowing when the body knows the area is clean and then instigates the formation of a scab. Genius.

Most people rush to clean the blood away because the first instinct is to stop the blood pouring out. I understand that need. However, rather than race to clean the area, simply *pause* and allow the body to do what it innately does best—heal. Be the observer of the healing process. We have also taught our children about the healing properties of their own saliva. Awhile ago our daughter cut her finger. I went through the steps with her I outlined above— blood, debris, scab, healing time —but I *also* reminded her of the healing properties of her own saliva. Sound crazy? It's not. Have your child lick their own wound, and no, they don't have to swallow their blood, they can spit it out. A person's own saliva serves a far greater purpose than merely the beginning point of immunity and digestion. Saliva is a powerful wound healer. Take a look at animals, domestic or wild—you'll see that they lick their own wounds. The saliva forms a seal, much like a sticky plaster. If you lick the back of your hand and then blow across your hand lightly you will feel a film across the surface; it will become slightly sticky and a little bit tight as well. That is the healing layer of your saliva.

At the age of ten when my mum popped the pill from the packet, filled a glass of water and slid it across the kitchen bench towards me confidently saying *'there you go, darling, this will make you feel better,'* it could have planted a belief that I required something from outside of my body to heal me and make me feel better. It could have planted a belief that I was incapable of healing, that indeed I must be incomplete in some way. I said no to the amoxicillin my mum had bought at the pharmacy and decided to go to my room, lie on my bed and rest. From that day my life was changed *forever.* I rarely as a child told my parents about a 'sickness' I was experiencing and I limited my coughing in front of my mum!

I was given an opportunity that day to test what my dad had taught me about trust and I grabbed that opportunity. I began my journey, slowly but surely, of understanding my body. I imagine most people don't have an opportunity like the one I was given: encouragement to question, and pearls of wisdom at a young age that help correct the course of my life path.

Instead ...

People approach **health like a recipe, followed diligently, unaltered, not questioned and handed down from generation to generation,** *done that way because that is the way it has always been done.*

Ah ha!

* How were you taught health? What were you taught about health?

* Were you taught that the body can heal some things and not others?

* Did someone at your school give you a class on health? What did they say?

* What are your demonstrated actions when you or your child 'get sick' or hurt themselves?

* What language are you using to portray health to yourself, those around you and your child?

* Are you simply 'doing' what you have always done?

Resources

'Got a cut? Lick your wound.'
www.VitalMoms.com/healthillusion

CHAPTER 9

The Health Illusion

'If they can get you asking the wrong questions,
they don't have to worry about answers.'

—— Thomas Pynchon

In order to understand health and the health illusion we must first reflect on this question 'where does health come from?'

There are two ways to answer:

> 1) Health comes to you from the outside-in, e.g. you go to someone to get something to take something away (Action: surrender responsibility). If you're feeling fine you are healthy. You go to someone when something is deemed to be wrong.

> 2) Health is created by you from the inside-out, you are an active participant in your health expression and you understand that you create every opportunity—good *and* bad—for the experience it affords you. You want to be your best you and you work towards reaching your optimum health potential (Action: self responsibility).

I imagine, like me, you were taught from a young age that health is defined by your feelings, the food you eat and your fitness. In other words if you are feeling good, eating well and moving a little you were deemed healthy. Our family health approach growing up was to reach for something to take something away, whatever that was—blood, cough, sore stomach etc so that once again I could 'feel fine'. My family very much sat in the first answer provided above where there is no expression of health, but rather a suppression of health; where taking something to mask the internal communication of my body went against what the very signs and symptoms were designed to do: to alert me to the 'messages' of importance, in a hierarchical manner.

But back than it was all about feelings, food and fitness. Of course this belief was founded on 'untruths'. The truth is that the signs and symptoms you experience don't 'just happen'. You don't wake up one morning and find you're living in Harry Potter's world and someone is waving a magic wand, saying today you will have a skin rash 'poof' and so you do, or a cough, a heart attack, a convulsion, a car crash. That world is untrue.

The truth is you perceive and sense the world around you via your nerve system. In response you create your own unique set of signs and symptoms within a body that is *working in your favour; working for you* to make sure you are expressing health to your highest level; to the best of your ability. It's your choice and the signs and symptoms are your creation.

There is some internal communication occurring prior to the 'popping up' of a symptom. This internal communication occurs between one's innate intelligence and one's educated mind. Together they create the focused and specific symptom or symptoms to be consciously experienced by you, the person creating it. It didn't 'just happen'. It may appear to be a situation of 'I was just bending over and then couldn't move' or 'I just woke up and felt _____' scenario, however it's not.

A symptom has a guided process of expression centered around the 3Ts—thoughts, trauma and toxins. Everybody's health path (newborns to the elderly), adaptation to life and symptom expression is created according to their perceptions of the world around them. Their world is sensed, filtered and experienced via their nerve system. Simply put ... a person's body and inherent health expression cannot be compared to another person; it is not age discriminatory and it's as unique as your figure print.

Take a look at the diagram below called 'The health illusion'.

The Health Illusion

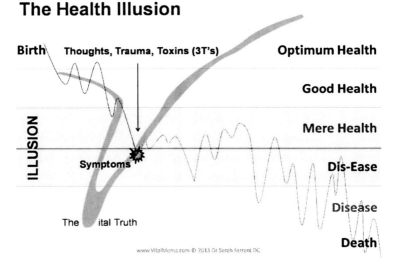

www.VitalMoma.com © 2013 Dr Sarah Farrant DC

Because the majority of people believe life is not in their control— that it is simply 'happening' to them —they expect their life's health journey to go from the top left to the bottom right over 'X' period of time—whatever that is.

The majority of people also *expect to be taking medications* when they begin the transitory journey to death, in fact people at that stage on average are consuming five medications in a bid to squash the feelings and their innate communication pathways.

This is pharmacology at its best—you're addicted, and they're making money.

I created the diagram you see here in a bid to nudge, and I hope enhance, your understanding of health. Let's see if I can do that!

It would appear from the diagram that people spend a short period of time in the top left, a good portion of time around the middle line and a long period of time in the bottom right, masking whatever's been created in a desperate bid to get back above the middle line again.

You can spend more of your life above the line if you take the time to look closely at how you are interpreting health, acknowledge where it comes from and take the necessary steps to alter your lifestyle to be more supportive of the way you want to live. I want you to live the longest period of your life, not your shortest, *well above* the line ... not *just* above the line. This doesn't mean that you will never die, it simply means that the quality of your life will be different. **The level of health you are currently experiencing is proportional to the way in which you interpret health.**

Let's take a closer look.

Every person is born with one hundred per cent optimum health potential. Period. This potential is not discriminatory against age, sex, colour, or religious and political alignment. It is present to be used as you see fit. From birth to death you create opportunities to nudge you in different directions and awaken yourself to your internal communication and its relationship with the world around you. These opportunities are created by yourself via the 3Ts—Thoughts,

Trauma and Toxins or, said another way, physical, chemical and emotional opportunities. Because they are created by you, you have the ability to change them. However most people believe they're not the captain of their ship nor the master of their destiny and hence do not change that which they have created. This is due to the indoctrinated system they were raised in (including myself) which defines health as feelings, food and fitness and the absence of signs and symptoms; an illusion within itself. Eighty-five per cent of the health challenges we see, hear and read about today are lifestyle-driven via the 3Ts. This means that because you created them via the life you were leading, you can change them by changing how you live. Simple.

However most people don't because;

1) they don't know how, or

2) they are too scared to because it means changing, or

3) they simply don't want to.

Let's face it: it's much easier for you to 'pop a pill' and continue living as you always have than to take the time to really understand your body's communication and make the internal shifts. People want to be healthy without the self-responsibility associated with it.

Umm.

So … life goes along and because you're 'feeling fine' you don't change any of your lifestyle and you now go from expressing optimum health to expressing good health. Life stills moves forward and challenges continue to be created via the 3Ts, however you're still not expressing signs and symptoms yet and so you continue to participate in life the way you always have and move from good health to mere health… and you're still 'feeling fine'. This is an insidious process which is different for everyone. Suddenly out of nowhere you 'got' a symptom, it supposedly just appeared with no conscious thought as to why. You woke up and now have 'x', 'y' and/or 'z'. You are now experiencing 'Dis-ease'. Dis-ease was coined by DD Palmer to mean a lack of ease within the body, 'things' not functioning, not coordinating as they should do or ought to. Because you define health as 'how you feel' you decide to do as you have always done without question and go to someone to get something to take something away. You consume what was prescribed for you, your symptoms go away, and you're now expressing 'mere health' and 'feeling fine'. You deem yourself to be healthy once again.

That is a health illusion.

You continue to live as you have always lived and ignore this opportunity to change an aspect of your life so your health can express differently. In taking the medication you 'pop' back above the line, continue living as you always have and as a result only express 'mere health'. You don't fulfill your potential of heading towards 'good health' and 'optimum health'. Masking the symptom and defining health as 'feeling fine' goes against what your body is innately and intelligently communicating to you. One way to well and truly 'shut the symptom up' is to dampen the innate internal neurological (nerve) communication network; the master communicating system.

After a period of time, again different for everyone, your body creates another symptom in response to the first symptom you suppressed with medications, which plummets you below the line and once again you're expressing 'dis-ease'. You return to the allopathic approach for another diagnosis and more medications. You dutifully oblige and take the medications, however this time when you 'pop' back up above the line you are not there for long. You're now on up to three different medications all masking the ones that came before the current one you are taking, with no sign of giving them up. You continue popping the pills, deciding to soldier on. You return to the allopathic approach for more medication to now mask the next symptom your body afforded you and as a result drop from dis-ease to disease where you are now expressing specific symptoms of a specific disease. You are now on up to five different medications. Your memory of what you took the first medication for is a distant one; what you do remember is that you are still taking 'that' medication. Your body's function begins to alter drastically due to the masking and dampening of your innate internal communication network and slowly but surely your transition to death begins. That is the life path of the average human being who lives the health illusion; the illusion that health is given to you via an outside-in process—an allopathic approach filled with pills and surgery. It's all based on how you feel.

When you buy into health being about 'FEElings' there is a 'fee' that comes with it; a price you pay. The fee is not only the price for the plethora of medications you end up on; it's your life.

I know there is another path you can take to live more of your life above the line than below it.

I know because I am living proof of it. I have not been to a medical doctor in almost three decades, my children were all born at home and have not been given nor offered over-the-counter or prescription medication, nor are they vaccinated or have they been to 'see' a medical doctor.

There are other, safer ways to approach health that keeps you well and away from the fee paying health illusion that most sit in. Knowing the safer ways will keep yourself and your family FUNctioning well and put the 'fun' back in your lives! To understand the safer way to approach health also means 'undoing' the years of living in an indoctrinated health system that keeps you living a life below the line and addicted to medications. Big Pharma prospers; you lose.

The first step towards living a different life is understanding what health is and who really is in control of it. To take this step let's first acknowledge that your nerve system is the master communicating system of your body. It is what you use to sense your world. Sensing your world via your nerve system gives you the opportunity to influence your physiology which, in turn, affects how you FUNction. Your level of health is directly related to how well you function. Your physiology is altered via the 3Ts—which you are in control of—in order to create the signs and symptoms to alert you to how you are participating in your life. Genius. You have at your internal disposal various mechanisms that assist you in the creation of your unique signs and symptoms, e.g. a homeostatic feedback loop, innate intelligence which governs the body and gives it life without you needing to consciously be aware of it (e.g. heart beating, cells cleaning, digestion, elimination etc) and your perceptions of the world around you. All are unique to you.

You can do one of two things from birth: 1) mask the symptoms (or have someone mask them for you) and you now know how that turns out or 2) you can work with your internal communication network, your nerve system, with the knowledge that you are a self-healing, self-regenerating and self-regulating person who is constantly adapting to their environment. When adaptation is challenged via the 3Ts (thoughts, trauma and toxins), symptoms are created to alert you. Indeed the symptoms are working with you, not against you. Acknowledging the 3Ts as external stressors that instigate changes within yourself will alert you to understanding more about how you are approaching your life and how well you are expressing health.

When I first looked to the nerve system I wanted the experience. I didn't want the facts and figures *about* the nerve system, I wanted to have an experience within my body that I would be able to connect with from a functional perspective. Randall, my boyfriend at the time (husband now), had been referred to a chiropractor by a member of the gym where we both worked. We went there with trepidation, unsure about what they would do and, of course, we had tucked inside our mind our illusionary health definition—feelings, food and fitness and health comes to you from something outside of yourself. Although we both were not into medications or drugs of any kind we did see a naturopath and would always leave with a new brew (tincture) of some sort. So entering into this 'what would they know' world came with a lot of judgement and a hearsay understanding of what 'they'—the chiropractors—do. Needless to say, I was blown away by their knowledge of the human body, their caring, their attitude to health and life and their love for what they did and gave to people. I left very humbled and booked myself in for an appointment as we left. I have never looked back.

When you decide that your life is in your hands, things change. As Joseph Campbell once said, 'Doors open where there previously weren't any doors.' You begin to see and experience life in ways other people cannot or do not want to see or experience. Your health takes on a whole new meaning and your approach to it is altered forever. (See Chapter 10: Health Approaches)

You can utilise and harness the power of your own nerve system for health expression and experience a different life. You can spend more of your life above the line. Period. You can choose to be an active participant in your own life and ask yourself different questions to come to different conclusions about your health and life. You can take responsibility for the decisions you have made and will make in the future and choose 'not to be fixed' and enjoy a life without drugs. In taking responsibility for your life and understanding the

power of the 3Ts and the unique symbiotic relationship they play
with your body in creating symptoms, you choose to look within to
fine tune your life to express your life's potential. Health is just one
aspect of that potential.

Beautiful.

 Ah ha!

FUNctional facts to assist with educating your kids[1]:

* The nerve system is a complex structure full of neurons
  (individual nerves) that transmit messages around the body
  to coordinate its actions. It's your body's electrical wiring.

* The nerve system has two parts, 1) a central nerve system
  (CNS—brain and spinal cord) which is protected by bone
  (skull and vertebrae) and 2) a peripheral nerve system
  (PNS—everything else outside of the central nerve system).
  The PNS connects the CNS to outside areas of the body.

* There are twelve nerves that branch from the brain. These
  are called cranial nerves and there are thirty-one pairs of
  nerves called spinal nerves that branch out from either side
  of the vertebra of the spinal column.

* Neurons quickly and precisely send signals as electrochemi-
  cal waves along axons to other cells. There are two types of
  neurons: sensory neurons and motor neurons.

* Sensory neurons change light, touch and sound into neural
  signals which are sent back to our CNS to help our body
  understand and adapt to its surroundings.

* Motor neurons transmit neural signals to activate muscles
  or glands.

Ah ha!

FUNctional facts (continued):

* There are approximately 100 billion neurons in the human brain and 13.5 million neurons in the human spinal cord. Incredible.

* The nerve system can transmit signals at speeds of 100 metres (328 feet) per second.

* The nerve system is the master communicating system in the body. It creates the changes to how we function based on how we respond our world via the 3Ts.

* The 3Ts are Thoughts (emotions), Trauma (physical) and Toxins (chemicals).What did they say?

Resources

'The magnificent you.'
www.VitalMoms.com/healthillusion

CHAPTER 10

Health Approaches

*'You must learn a new way to think before
you can master a new way to be.'*
—— Marianne Williamson

The three health approaches flooded my mind as I was going through our CYFS saga. I wanted to prove a point: the 'system' I was thrust into and what they knew about health was exceptionally limited and different to mine. It forced me to see how I could indeed *organise the worlds health information into bite-sized pieces so people could understand it* and form a succinct system for the everyday person to understand that was irrefutable when you 'saw it' and became educated on it.

I believe what you will read here will begin to unravel some of the confusion out there about health, what it is and where it comes from. This section will afford you an opportunity to step outside the current dogmatic approach to health which states that if you're 'sick' you go to someone to get something to take something away.

It's time to debunk that myth and share the truth.

During this chapter I will introduce you to three different health approaches. Health approaches and health professions are not interchangeable words. My reasoning and philosophy may be in contrast to your current views and beliefs about health and where it comes from, or it may not. It might be the validity you have been looking for or an epiphany you did not expect. In either event, I ask that you place your opinions to the side and read like a child of twelve who has just found out something for the first time—with excitement, anticipation and 'Ah ha!' moments. For if I have not ruffled your feathers, caused you to think differently or enabled your mind to be expanded then I have not done what I set out to do!

Here goes …

When you consider the different health approaches available to you, there really are just three. I'm sure right now you are jumping up and down saying 'Three? There are way more than three!' And yes, there are more than three health *professions* but not more than three health *approaches*.

There is a difference.

As you read you will see how, today, society has placed so many health professions in a pot and mixed them all together so you, the consumer, find it hard to distinguish who does what, based on what the beliefs of that profession are and what approach to health they are using. Two of the health professions I will mention here are the antithesis of each other in their approach *and* philosophy and the rest, well, they pretty much sit in a mixed pot according to how they are grouped together. (See Chapter 11: Are you a Health Slider?)

Understanding the philosophical backgrounds of the three health approaches will begin to unravel for you why today's society is so confused by so many conflicting ideas about health and where it comes from. However, if you take the time to understand these approaches then you gain power over your health choices, confident in the decision you make and ultimately become a 'health slider' moving between the three approaches when *you choose* to do so. Essentially, you're empowered!

As I move through the three health approaches I want you to consider where you currently sit. Are you making your health decisions and your family's health decisions from one approach? Are you using two or even all three of them?

Let's first take a look at the picture given here.

What do you see?

Some of you who have been to my live presentations or viewed an online video of mine will pick it right away so this shall be easy and a nice reminder. But for those of you new to me ... what do you see?

Do you see a woman? Yes? Do you see two women? Yes?

If you said yes to seeing two women you would be right! In this picture there

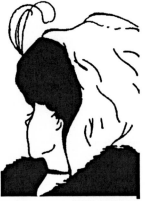

W. E. Hill, 1915

is an image of a young woman and an image of an old woman. The challenge is being able to see them both ... freely flicking between the two.

If you can only see one woman you probably have no idea that another one exists other than I told you there are two images, or you might have known that another completely different view of a women existed in the image however you simply couldn't see it. Your demonstrated behavior was likely one of frustration because you're blind to the other woman or you dismissed it and didn't believe me when I said there was a different view of a woman in the image. However it's usually not until someone takes but a moment to point out what it looks like and outlines the defining boundaries of it for you that suddenly it 'pops' out and you notice it. Because you see it you're unable to NOT see it. Now you effortlessly flick between the two views in the one image.

It's the same in health. The overall image we are looking at is health and the two different views of the woman represent the different approaches—only in health, there are three approaches.

When you predominately approach health in one way you generally have no idea or are naive to other approaches existing; you're blind to anything but the most common approach you use. Essentially then you only see one woman. It's only when 1) you begin educating yourself on the different approaches, which is usually initiated by asking different questions; 2) you're open to someone in your community by virtue of the conversation you are having or 3) you're tired of doing the same thing over and over again, expecting a different result that doesn't come, that you than decide to look elsewhere.

I was introduced to this image when I was studying psychology and it has always stuck with me when I'm contemplating different points of view; a nice reminder that there is a series of concurrent 'things' occurring at the same time in your life. In using this image as a metaphor for your health you can understand that there is more than one way approach health, with some approaches occurring concurrently. Unless we ask ourselves different questions to see a different way we wouldn't know that it was happening. Another principle you could draw from this image is that if you are only seeing the old way, the traditional way (old woman: allopathic) then you're unaware that there are other health approaches with distinct and different philosophies that exist (young woman: alternative, alternate)—that are established, scientific, credible, and successful in and of themselves.

But in order to see these other ways to health and experience them you have to first begin with asking yourself different questions. When you begin asking different questions, different doors open and you will experience a whole new health world. I've personally utilised all three of the health approaches through my life. When we were going through the CYFS saga I was this open vessel into which information about health was flowing—namely the different health approaches. I found I couldn't stop writing, wanting to share with people the different ways to look at health, helping them to reach different conclusions about what health is and how we express it, ultimately keeping themselves and their child safe in an ever changing 'sick care' world ... it was pouring out of me.

I knew I had to get my material organised if I was to share it successfully. So I began with the names for each health approach and decided to start with what I knew growing up—the allopathic approach. And being a self-confessed word nerd, I examined where these words came from. I was stunned at what I found.

I looked up AlloPATHIC: where **Pathic** from L. *pathicus*, from Gk. *Pathikos* 'remaining passive'[3]

Oh my gosh, I thought. I'm onto something here.

Okay what did I 'use' next ...

I wrote down 'Complementary and Alternative Medicine' because that was where I went after exiting the allopathic approach. I went digging and found that AlterNATIVE: where **Native (n.)** 1838 'the other of two which may be chosen,'[4] means 'offering a choice.'[5] Again, I wasn't disappointed!

I was knuckle biting by this time.

Off I set to look closely at the allopathic and the alternative health approaches by reviewing what they both offered to people. I thought about my own experiences in addition to the philosophy, language, beliefs, clothing, systems, health interpretation, roles, involvement, personal authority, etc. I started to bullet point my observations into either the allopathic or the alternative bucket. As I divided the points I noted there were a number of points that simply didn't 'fit in' or make sense when attributed to either the allopathic or alternative approaches. So I thought there must be a third approach where there were traditionally only two—allopathic and alternative. I hunted and hunted for a word that would flow on from the two I already had. I knew I wanted the word to start with 'A' so it would be easy for people to remember. I combed the dictionary until 'Bingo!' I found it. 'Alternate' where 'nate' means 'inborn'.

Suddenly before my eyes I had a system.

I respect that **ALL three approaches are different. All three are represented in society; all three are needed** and because of this it's wise to see the three joined like a triangle with health centered in the middle and, as the consumer, you get to choose where you enter the triangle. I had *created a system to organise the world's health information into bite-sized pieces so people could understand it* and have the opportunity to become a 'health slider'; empowered to make the best health choice for themselves and their children.

I was excited and I had work to do!

What follows is a brief description of the major points in each health approach. They are given below in order of how they came into my life.

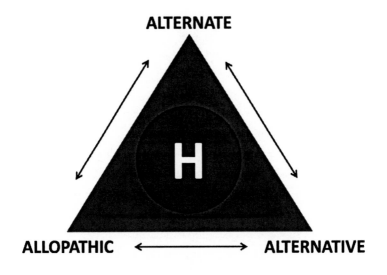

The health arena
©2014 VitalMoms.com

The AlloPATHIC Approach (mechanism, medicine)

I was raised in the allopathic approach and I suspect you may have been too. I also come from a lineage of family members who are medical doctors. In hindsight what I recall from being a consumer of the allopathic approach was that I was kept passive in my 'search' for health.

Do you remember the story of my mum and I in the kitchen—the one when I coughed a few times and she zoomed me to our family medical doctor? I've mentioned it a few times because it illustrates so many interesting points. Here are some of the main ideas I observed and experienced within this health approach:

- It keeps you passive: 'pathic' means ... 'remaining passive'.
- It teaches you to surrender responsibility to someone else.

- It's not your fault: The allopathic approach suggests you are either lucky or unlucky and that *life is happening to you*. Life is seen as a random set of events that you have no hand in shaping nor control over. You therefore are not the captain of your ship nor are you the master of your destiny. 'That's just life' as the saying goes and it is not your fault. This lets you off the 'self-responsibility hook'.

- It's about fear and 'what if' situations: Health decisions are made from fear and 'what if' situations: 'What's going to happen if you don't take it?', 'What if something gets worse?', 'What if this doesn't go away?' What if, what if, what if …

- It's a quick fix: The allopathic approach has you looking for a 'quick fix'. You define health by how you feel and as such when you are not feeling fine you want 'X' feeling removed so once again you feel like the 'normal' you. You go to someone to get something to take something away.

- Health comes from the outside-in; you are only the sum of your parts: Essentially the hierarchy of your body in an allopathic approach to health goes from systems to organs to tissues to cells to organelles to molecules to atoms, stop. That's how the body is made up. In acknowledging you as the sum of your parts the allopathic approach can justify producing individual medications for the individual areas of your body—head, throat, heart, shoulder, lungs, bowels, skin etc. The smallest component of the human body according to this approach is the atom of which no further division can take place. There is a belief that there is no intelligence within the atom and this is why this approach relies on something outside of you (drugs or surgery) to remove the symptoms so once again you experience health based on how you define it—feelings.

- Disease must be fought: It is believed that disease enters you from the outside and, because you didn't create it, it has to be fought and/or removed by cutting it out, slicing it out, dicing it out, burn it out, draw it out and so forth. Bottom line ... disease must be fought and gotten rid of.
- Health is about how you feel: The only way to define health is by feelings, food and fitness.

The allopathic approach comes from an OUTSIDE-IN approach to health.

Let's move on to the approach I moved to next ...

The AlterNATIVE Approach

Any profession that is not dispensing drugs or medications of any kind is placed in the Alternative or more widely known Complementary and Alternative Medicine (CAM) bucket where 'NATIVE' means 'offering a choice'. My reflection of this approach began to get very interesting as I was attempting to make sense of why health approaches were called what they were called. Interestingly, when I'm speaking around the world and ask people what they think 'alternative' means, they usually respond with 'natural', 'whole', 'organic' or 'of the earth,' but the truth is it means 'offering a choice'.

This approach contains the largest 'bucket' of health *professions*.

Professions that have collectively been placed in the CAM 'bucket' include naturopathy, osteopathy, chiropractic, Chinese medicine, aromatherapy, Reiki, massage and many more. These individual health professions acknowledge there is a special something, an energy, governing the body. Some professions call it Prana, Chi, Qi, Ki, Innate, Life Force, Pneuma, Num, and Mana.

However ... because of the inherent need to be 'the one' (re-read Chapter 11: Are You a Health Slider?), and obtain the 'top dog' position, these CAM professions began to morph and adopt similarities to that of the health approach sitting in the 'top dog' position—the allopathic approach—which leaves you confused about who does what. Processes, language, identities, clothing, systems, and philosophical beliefs all insidiously change to the allopathic approach. I kept at the forefront of my mind *complementary to* and *alternative from*—medicine. Interesting isn't it? And when I looked at it like this it was easy to see why it was simpler for people to move from the allopathic approach to the alternative approach than it was to move from the allopathic approach to the alternate approach. The alternative approach looks similar to the allopathic approach and thus poses little threat.

The mechanistic philosophy that drives the allopathic approach has infiltrated the alternative (CAM) approach; even though the professions within the alternative approach are different, their governing approach is the same. People who are on the way out of the allopathic approach find the alternative approach a safe place to move to: it looks the same, feels the same, they speak a similar language and provide something to take something away, again where being symptom-free means you're healthy again. So for all intents and purpose, it is the same, minus the laboratory-made medications, dispensing of drugs and performance of surgery.

Here are the lead bullet points of the alternative CAM approach:

- You go to someone, to get something, to take something away however, now you have a vast number of different health *professions* to chose from in order to get what you want to take 'X' away;

- You remain passive in your pursuit of health;

- Someone is still telling you what is wrong with you;

- Fear remains at the fore and 'what if' situations continue to be determined;

- You remain the sum of your parts; a specific 'remedy' is supplied for your symptoms;
- You continue to be told disease is something that comes from the outside-in and must be fought;
- Health continues to be defined by your FEElings—if you're symptom-free, you're healthy;

I asked the question, 'What separates the alternative from the allopathic?' I thought there must be more than simply drugs and surgery and what is given to the person to 'fix' what it is that they 'have'. I kept digging and found three:

> 1) An alternative health professional will make suggestions, rather than a diagnosis, per se;

> 2) Time is given to you to decide what you want to do about the suggested symptoms;

> 3) There is an acknowledgement of an *inner intelligence* that knows what to do and keeps you healthy, i.e. beats your heart, digests your food, creates bowel movements, secretes oils, sloughs your skin, blinks your eyes, etc.

Many a wise man has said **the quality of your life is based on the quality of your questions**. If you're asking the same questions then you will get the same response; however if you begin to ask different questions, you begin to open new doors and start to see things in a different way.

Do you remember the chapter where I honed in on how health is being defined both by society and the dictionary? The one where I shared I went to the local shopping mall to ask anybody who would stop what they thought health was? Do you remember the responses I got?

Here they are again:

1) Health is having no signs & symptoms;

2) Health is having no pain;

3) Health is eating well;

4) Health is about exercising; and

5) Health is about being happy.

Do you remember the definition I shared from Dorland's Pocket Medical Dictionary, the WHO and the chiropractic profession? They say health is:

'optimum physical, mental and social wellbeing and

not necessarily the absence of disease and infirmity.'

Two vastly different ways to look at health, wouldn't you say? One is about feeling, food and fitness and the other is about function and living an optimum life with and without disease.

This leads me to the alternate approach.

The AlterNATE Approach (vitalism, chiropractic)

This is the life and health approach I sit in alongside my husband. It is the approach we are choosing to raise our children with. All of our children were born at home, the last of which was a breech (See Chapter 17: Ups and Downs of Pregnancy and Birth). I didn't read books or subscribe to a particular way to birth. What I had was what was taught to me at the age of seven—TRUST. Trust that I had the answers within me; trust that I am a self-healing, self-regenerating and self-regulating organism who is constantly adapting to my environment; trust that my child has intelligence and that he/she will know what to do—instinctively and intuitively. As a result of my trust in who I am, I didn't partake in the medicalisation of pregnancy with its ultrasounds, internal examinations, blood work, vaccinations and so forth that keep people in an allopathic 'fear based' and 'what if' approach to health.

Our children have never had a medication—over the counter or prescription and have not been to a medical doctor. It is this approach, as I mentioned right at the beginning, that is the antithesis of the allopathic approach. This approach realises when two things are alike something is not needed, hence the positioning in stark contrast to the allopathic approach. To embrace this approach takes a paradigm shift in one's thinking. There is no disguise here, no attempt to be like 'the one', no attempt to tell people what is wrong with them, but rather a respect for the capabilities of the human body and the intelligence that lives within—physically, chemically and emotionally.

Here are the lead points of this approach:

- The nerve system is acknowledged as the master communicating system and any interference to the nerve system creates different states of health expression;

- People are active participants in creating their health;

- People look for change rather than a 'fix it';

- Responsibility and accountability are accepted not avoided;

- The body expresses perfect order rather than random chaos;

- Health is wholeness; the whole body is considered and the interconnectedness acknowledged;

- People create health expressions as opposed to being 'sick';

- There is the acknowledgement of an inner intelligence which is specifically referred to as innate intelligence; and

- Health is about how you FUNction.

You will see, as you read on, that the beliefs and philosophy of the alternate approach are different to the alternative approach and in stark contrast to the allopathic approach.

One health profession that sits comfortably in this health approach is the chiropractic profession, the largest health profession in the world using no drugs or surgery. Those who use the alternate approach to health and life acknowledge that within the universe there exists a perfect order; a balanced order. We see this order within the universe—high tides and low tides, males and females, sunrises and sunsets, construction and destruction, light and dark, famine and obesity and so on.

If we take this understanding into the body we see the balance that exists there also—toxic and tonic reactions occurring at the exact same time, sodium and potassium pumps across cellular membranes occurring at the exact same time and cell growth and cell death occurring at the exact same time. In fact, we can say one is positive (e.g. tonic reactions, sodium pump, cell growth) and the other one negative (e.g. toxic reactions, potassium pump and cell death). The take-home message here is that there exists balance. Our experiences, positive and negative, are occurring at the exact same time; indeed you cannot have one without the other.

People who use this approach see life as their own creation; they have the power and the wherewithal to impact it in any way they choose, in fact their life to date has been a result of the choices they made along the way and the remainder of their life will be based on the decisions they make in the future. Life is not happening to them. They are the captain of their ship and a master of their destiny.

As such, people are active participants in their health creation and respond well when questions are framed from a perspective of trust and their noted ability to change. They are not searching for health because they understand that it is not missing. Rather they choose to express health in a different way, enabling them to ask different questions, leading them to different conclusions which alters the decisions and choices they make.

People in this approach acknowledge themselves as a self-healing, self-regenerating and self-regulating organism that is constantly adapting to the environment. They also understand that the power that made the body (innate) heals the body and their health is non-linear, forever fluctuating and rarely stagnant. At the core is a strong philosophical belief that there is a direct relationship between your body's structure and how you function, and that how you function has a direct relationship with your nerve system, the master communicating system of your body. Any interference to the nerve system—physically, chemically and/or emotionally—will affect your growth, adaptation, transformation and, of course, how you function.

Okay, let's look at the hierarchy of the body. Under this alternate approach there are many levels.

Ready? Here we go …

Systems, organs, tissues, cells, organelles, molecules, atoms (remember this is where the allopathic approach stops!), subatomic particles, vibrations, energy and light. Light, when we break it down further, creates a positive and a negative charge.

The Buddhists say;

'We'll teach them the illusion until they are ready for the truth.'

Are you ready for the truth?

The truth is your body exists with both health and disease (positive and negative); you cannot have one without the other. You are the master of your destiny, and you choose your level of health expression.

Choosing what health approach is right for you and your family is challenging enough and part of choosing is making sure you understand *how* health is approached. By outlining each of these approaches for you, you now have the option of seeing where to use them. I use the alternate approach; it is where I am most comfortable. I have used all three of these approaches at some point in time through my life. I was raised in the allopathic approach and began at a young age to move away from it—it just didn't make sense to me. Chiropractic was not in my life at that stage and so my next best option was the alternative approach to health. I stayed here for some time until I was inspired by Ken and Karen to become a chiropractor. I haven't looked back.

All three health approaches are necessary because they all exist. Where you want them entering your family's health is your choice and discussed in the next chapter.

 Ah ha!

* Are you making your health decisions and your family's health decisions from one approach?
* Are you using two, or even all three, of them?
* Do you trust that you and your child have everything to express health?

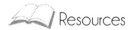 Resources

'Health approach quick reference guide'
www.VitalMoms.com/healthillusion

CHAPTER 11

Are You a Health Slider?

*'We cannot solve our problems with the same
level of thinking that created them.'*

—— Albert Einstein

One principle of health YOU MUST KNOW ... however only a handful of people do.

At college I missed out on receiving the prestigious 'Virgil Strang Philosophy Award' and I haven't gotten over it but I've moved on. People at college would recognize me as a student who LOVED philosophy as it afforded me the opportunity to question, explore, discover and interpret a world according to me. It was awesome. I certainly honor and entertain the thought of being a philosopher however I must admit to myself I cannot compare to the incredible thinkers who came before me. I prefer to see myself and my life as one big gigantic 'Socratic think tank'!

My dad was the epitome of Socratic enquiry—question after question to get me to the truth of what I wanted an answer for, stimulating my own critical thought and illuminating my ideas so

I could come to my own conclusion. Without this type of thought process and my systemised mind I wouldn't have been able to come to the conclusions I have, and the wonderful health teachings offered would at best be energetic thoughts drifting in the ether.

For many years I thought about the principle of *the one and the many and the many and the one* and wondered how it could be attributed to health. There was something inherent in this principle that sang to me when I came across it many moons ago. At the time I had no idea what song that was other than I knew it could be attributed to health; how to do that I wasn't yet clear on. So I let it lie dormant for awhile—well, a long while—percolating in the back of my mind with no real understanding for how I could use it to educate the public … until I went through the CYFS saga. During this time it became very clear how this powerful principle could be used as a teaching point in health.

Before I dive into this principle it will be necessary to reiterate from the previous chapter what I mean when I use the words 'health profession/s' and 'health approaches'. They are NOT interchangeable words. When I mention 'health profession' I'm referring to a collective bundle of health professions (e.g. naturopathy, osteopathy, homeopathy, Chinese medicine, Reiki, aromatherapy, massage, etc.) or I'm referring singularly to one (e.g. medicine, allopathy). When I mention 'health approach' I am referring to the philosophical alignment in which the health profession defines health and educates people regarding health and *presents themselves to the public*. You will understand more as you read on.

Understanding how this principle plays out in the health arena will have a major impact on how you view health. It's subtle, yet has a big impact. Understanding it will enable you to become a 'health slider'. I hear you saying to yourself 'Health slider? What is that?'

Well, let me explain …

A 'health slider' is someone who can seamlessly move between the three health *approaches* with a solid awareness of:

1) The three health *approach*es

2) Which health professions sit in what health approach

3) Their own responsibility when choosing what to use as a consumer of health and a participant in life.

A 'health slider' has the knowledge, confidence and trust to choose what approach they want to use and when. A health slider is a well-educated individual who acts in an aware manner and takes full responsibility for their life. A health slider is well aware of the principle *the one and the many and the many and the one.*

A 'health slider' understands the difference between the health approaches to be as follows:

- Allopathic: trauma/emergency care

- Alternative: trauma/emergency care and by many for day-to-day health

- Alternate: utilised in day-to-day health for optimal health function from birth to death however it is also used in trauma/emergency care

If you're new to my work, the principle of 'the one and the many and the many and the one' will be new to you as well. If you want to make changes to your current health circumstance and embrace different ways to view, approach and interpret health then this is an essential and important principle to understand. To begin sifting through all the confusion out there about what health is, how we 'get it', where it comes from and, more importantly, being able to identify what health philosophy a particular profession aligns itself with (which in turn has an impact on their approach) you must consider this piece, the principle of *the one and the many and the many and the one.*

Think of it like this …

When you are *the one*, you want, need and/or require *the many* to follow you.

When you are part of *the many*, you want to be *the one* who people follow and look to for advice.

This principle is played out in two ways 1) via the health professions and where they want to be placed and 2) via the consumers and what they wish to 'see'.

Currently the allopathic profession (aka: medicine, mechanistic, medicinal where *pathic* means remaining passive) *is seen* to be *the one*—holding the power, the political connections, the purse strings and they have supposed credibility. No doubt you've noticed that this balance of power is beginning to cave and tip in a different direction. But, for now, they retain the 'top dog' position. As a result the 'almighty allopathic muscle' has been able to regulate, discredit (e.g. chiropractic other professions and organizations), deregister and defame individuals/groups/organizations and professions.

The bottom line is *when you are the one you want the many.* Interesting isn't it?

Let me share a lighter example of how this gets played out …

Let's say you are not yet in a relationship. You are part of the herds of people (the many) who are on their own, looking for the perfect partner to settle down with (the one). Eventually you find the one; you date for a period of time and then decide to get married. You are now no longer part of the herd (the many) looking for the one—quite the opposite, actually. Because you are now with 'the one' you begin casting your eye at 'the many'!

True … right? I know you're nodding! Read carefully this next piece—it's important…

If you look at preventative health you see a conglomerate of health *professions* which perhaps were instigated into society at their time as the next best to the allopathic *approach*. Many have maintained distinctions in their growth and development to position themselves in direct contrast to the allopathic community. Every health *profession* has principles to guide them: a philosophy, an art, an approach and a body of research.

But as humans, with an inherent wish 'to be the one' we began to see various health professions acknowledge the kudos the top health profession (allopathic *approach*) receives and so, in an attempt to be 'the one', many alternative and alternate health professions began selling out on their unique philosophy, their unique approach to health, their language, their dress, their systems, their beliefs and on and on—all in a bid to be like 'the one'. Health professions once established in direct contrast to the 'top dog' are now diluted in a bid to 'fit in', be like 'the one' in the hope of one day toppling the 'top dog'. It's a sad but true account of what has happened and what continues to be happening within health professions today.

You only have to look around to see how, as a consumer, you can be confused as you set about learning to identify and understand what different health professions stand for. **Most health consumers see the allopathic approach as the one to go to and as such have an underlying expectation that other health professions, even if they are 'alternative or alternate to' will have an element of the allopathic approach within them.**

The problem becomes: what happens when they don't?

Can you see how this confuses people and professions? It's an identity crisis of the health kind.

Let's look at it this way ...

Let's say you are wanting to move away from the allopathic approach to health, an approach you have used for years, for whatever reason that may be. Because of your upbringing and the indoctrinated health system used in your family—doing it that way because that is the way it has always been done; no questions asked— you exit your current and most well known health approach to find something different. The problem arises when looking for something else, because your interpretation, how you define health and what you expect other professions to be like has NOT CHANGED. In other words, when 'Alternative or Alternate' health *professions* don't have elements of the Allopathic *approach* (medicine) within them (philosophies, beliefs, language, look, systems, processes), rather than look at what the 'Alternative or Alternate' can offer, people end up, at best, misunderstanding them and at worse dismissing them.

People are heard saying, '_____ doesn't work'; '___ is quackery' and so forth.

Umm.

People then begin to discredit these other professions (not individuals but professions)—simply because people have chosen *not to see their differences and uniqueness* but rather have chosen to wonder why they are not like what society is used to. So it becomes for these other, or rather, different health professions, a double edged sword instigated by the underpinning of this subtle principle—*when you are the one you want the many and when you are part of the many you want to be the one.*

When it comes to the race between two similar professions for the top of the health pyramid, one thing holds true: the top position is like a vortex sucking in professions that are so needing and wanting to be like 'the one'. And who becomes confused? You, the consumer.

Curled inside this understanding of the 'one and the many' principle is a deep history—so deep that if you're not asking yourself different questions about health, you wouldn't notice it at all.

Understanding the philosophical backgrounds of the three health *approaches* will begin to unravel for you why today's society is bamboozled by so many conflicting ideas about health and where it comes from.

Where in your life have you dismissed/not returned to/thought twice about a health profession because they didn't 'look like', sound like or approach health in the way you were used to—the indoctrinated system, the allopathic way? What was it you were looking for that you didn't find?

Interestingly, when it comes to professions of alternative or alternate health, people often dismiss the whole profession if their experience, their process, the language wasn't similar to the one they were used to. I am not sure what they were expecting but if you enter anything new then by virtue of it being new, it will be different. Be open to the educational opportunity and what that profession's approach has to offer. For years I chose to label chiropractors as uneducated hair-brained quacks who 'crack you'. I bought into what I was being told by my parents, peers, TV, radio, print media, teachers, gym clients and other people in other health professions who simply didn't know the truth.

How wrong and how judgmental I was.

When I decided to lay aside my beliefs about what I thought health was and where it came from—as uncomfortable as that was—I began to embrace a TOTALLY DIFFERENT health path. Rather than me verbally labeling the chiropractic profession … I, as a chiropractor, became the subject of those labels. Interesting isn't it? You carry, don't you, your perceived ideas about what health is, judging, closed perhaps, scared to make a move because 'that' profession doesn't look, or behave like what you are used to.

 Ah ha!

- Where in your life have you dismissed/not returned to/ thought twice about a health profession because they didn't 'look like', sound like or approach health in the way you were used to—the indoctrinated system, the allopathic way perhaps?

- What was it you were looking for that you didn't find?

CHAPTER 12

Drug Pushers are Closer to Your Kids Than You Think!

'If drugs make you healthy, shouldn't the people taking the most drugs be the healthiest?'

I have been known to 'tell it like it is' and this chapter on 'Drug pushers' is going to be no different. I guarantee as you read through there will be shock as well as some 'Ah ha!' moments too. In order to understand how close the drug pushers really are you must have an awareness of how you are interpreting health and where you think it comes from or this chapter might see you 1) placing the book on your book shelf never to be picked up again 2) throwing it against a wall, outraged at the content or at worst 3) putting it in the bin! So please go back and re-read the chapters to help you understand what health is and where it comes from for you. Once you've done that … read on!

This is not a chapter for the fainthearted but rather one to alert you to the fact that drug pushers are closer to your kids than you may think. My purpose for writing this is to raise awareness and break the illusion that exists about who the initial drug pushers are and unveil a truth that not everyone wants to read, hear or acknowledge.

At no other time than in the 0-7 year age range will a child experience such rapid growth; neurologically and physically. Our senses are heightened because our language is limited. We rely on the actions demonstrated by those around us and the observations we make about those actions. Our neurons form connections about the actions we observe, thereby laying down a plethora of 'neurological experiences' to be drawn upon at a later time to assist us with interpreting our world. Children will, through this time, create opportunities to challenge their body in order to stimulate development. Discomfort and pain are one of the many signs which indicate that changes are taking place internally and growth is occurring. Children will create health challenges to grow, develop and adapt to their environment.

When children are young and have created a change in their health circumstance (e.g. a fever) parents want their children to be comforted. One of those ways is by wanting to take away the symptoms that you perceive them to 'have'. There are two ways in which to 'remove' the symptom 1) you go to someone to get something to take something away, leaving with a prescription which you then get filled or 2) you quickly drive to your local pharmacy to purchase an over-the-counter medication based on a self diagnoses of the 'symptom' they 'got'. Either way you return home with something to give to your child. Remember the example I shared about my mum and I being in the kitchen and what happened when I coughed a couple of times? My mum wanted to get something to take my symptom away.

Let me share this piece ... I feel it is important in case someone thinks I'm being unkind to my mum. I'm not. My mum did the best at raising my sister and I with the information that was available to her based on her own beliefs about what health was. These other approaches to health that I share are not new—they were there at the time she was parenting us and still there today—she just didn't see them because either she wasn't looking for anything different, she was asking the same questions or nobody took the time to challenge her on what she thought health was or educate her on what it could be. Mum did what the majority of the people at the time did because that's the way it's always been done. Mum's approach was based on her interpretation of health—feelings, food and fitness and so in a Pavlov's dog classic stimulus-response way she remained within her understanding that health is about how you feel. The drugs do their job ... you no longer feel what you were feeling ... you're now healthy. Period.

So that day when I was bundled into Mum's car and taken to Uncle Richard's to get some amoxicillin to 'nip my cough in the bud' I observed my mum do three things which became an anchor for my future reference:

    1) she panicked;

    2) raced, without second thought, to the allopathic approach; and

    3) we returned home with drugs ... *to give to me.*

Arriving home, Mum filled the glass of water, popped a pill from the pill packet, and while sliding the pill and the glass towards me over the kitchen bench said with a smile and a comforting voice 'There you go, darling, this will make you feel better'. This action, of course, began when I was very, very young.

Children often naturally shy away from medications *unless an association is created for them.* You often see images of children with closed mouths and a parent or health professional attempting to force a spoon with medicated liquid on it into their mouth. Because of their heightened senses and lack of a lexicon their smell is used as a defence for their body. They innately know what they are about to consume or receive will not be of benefit to the growth they are undertaking.

However, as a parent you are not 'seeing' health any differently to what was taught to you via the observations you made about *your* parents and their actions, so you 'soldier on' and force your child to swallow the liquid or receive whatever it maybe, even if it is a little. During the struggle you continue to say 'Oh darling, just a little—this will make you feel better,' and you keep saying it over and over again with each health challenge, spill or fall had; each situation being an opportunity to reinforce the message 'this will make you feel better' or 'this will help you,' whatever 'this' is: Band-Aid, mercurochrome, medicine, pill, tablet, cream, or injection. This firmly anchors a lifelong belief (if they don't choose to question health and where it comes from) that their body is not correct in creating the signs or symptoms it has and it's incapable of healing and growth and adapting to life. The lesson learnt for the child and the experience had is very clear: health comes from the outside-in which makes you 'feel better'. It establishes a dependence on something outside of them self to make them feel better, to make something that is not nice go away.

It's the parents who push the drugs and it all starts in the house.

I know it's hard 'to swallow' but it's true. Parents firmly establish the anchor via the lexicon used and the actions demonstrated in conjunction with the belief that the human body needs something outside of itself to remove the feelings— the symptoms—a person is experiencing. The end result is 'feeling good'.

Cut to … your child is now twelve years old. They appear to be enjoying school and their report card reads well. However, you begin to wonder where your once communicative child has gone. The teenage years have hit sooner than you thought and their world 'suddenly' is being shaped by their peers. No longer are they reaching out to you to assist with solving a problem they have. Their friends, 'Doctor Google' and electronic devices give them immediate non-threatening and supportive 'advice'. In every household that has children there is an arbitrary line that gets crossed; a line that appears at different ages. The age can vary, but children as young as twelve years start to replace the 'drug pusher' from the home with the 'drug pusher' in the school yard or on the street.

Children who choose drugs from the yard or a street 'drug pusher' do so as a way of escaping some kind of challenge and by virtue of their actions are deemed to be troubled children 'mixing with the wrong crowd'. But hang on … is it a wrong crowd or are they doing what they have been taught to do: if you have a problem, take something—it will make it go away.

Parents often become disillusioned about why their child took the drugs, but they're disillusioned only because they 'bought into' the health illusion in the first place.

A large portion of a parent's time and energy is then spent attempting to reverse the anchor and the lexicon that the parent firmly established in the first place, from birth. What was a *quick fix anchor* for taking away the symptoms when they were young then becomes a *quick fix answer* for taking away the challenge of a teenager and young adult.

Umm.

Little things when they are little turn into big things when they are bigger.

If, as a society we are so against illegal drugs, why then are we so supportive of over-the-counter and prescription medications?

Did you know ... 'annual deaths from painkillers now surpass those from heroin and cocaine combined, and have pushed the overall death toll from drugs above deaths from motor-vehicle crashes in some states [in the USA],' said R Gil Kerlikowske, Director of the White House office of National Drug Control Policy.

But that is just the tip of the iceberg ...

According to the American College of Preventative Medicine 'over the counter medication use in children is twice that of prescription medication.'[2] Why? Because it is easy to access, there are minimal laws that govern age and purchase and it's convenient to 'take the feelings away'.

As a parent you then get on this merry-go-round, not questioning what health is and why health challenges are created by an intelligent body in the first place. Rather, you're happy doing health this way because this is the way it has always been done. Then you're dumbfounded, pissed off, irritated and at worst angry that your child could be so stupid as to 1) 'try' an illegal addictive drug 2) 'try' a prescription drug handed out by a mate who says 'Try this; it helps me' 3) purchase a highly addictive over-the-counter drug or 4) accept a drug from a pusher on the street, all in a bid to make them feel better. It's simply demonstrated action you as a parent anchored and mirrored for them from a young age, indeed the first twelve years of their life.

Essentially you are confusing yourself and your child:

0-12 years: 'Here take this. It will make you feel better.'

+12 years: 'Why did you take that? It won't help you!'

Makes you wonder, doesn't it, what lies you've been told about health that perpetuate the myth of symptoms being bad, so you enter into a dependent medicated system that has you or your child become addicted and pharma making the profits.

You might be having an 'Ah ha' moment right now and you're quite possibly thinking 'Well, that is all well and good, Dr Sarah, but how can I change it?' If this is you, then great, because it means you're on your way to looking at health differently. I've put together some steps to consider to assist with making this transition to a different way of looking at health:

1) At the root of your own and / or your child's *health expression* (a term I coined to replace the word 'sickness') is their nerve system, the master communicating system of the body. The nerve system controls the communication between the brain and the body and back again. Nerve disturbance to the flow of messages diminishes the body's ability to express health. A child's perception and response to early health expressions (sickness) is crucial for their future. Your response to your child's health expression is even more crucial as it lays down a set of values and beliefs that they anchor to as a future way of responding to their health— good and bad. Making sure you educate yourself and your child on the capabilities of the human body is one of the best ways to boost their health potential.

2) Begin to firmly anchor a belief in your child that their body is complete and heals itself. Part of the healing opportunity is being aware of and noticing your body when it is in a comfortable state *and* when in an uncomfortable state. Teach them to trust in their ability to adapt to their environment. Create the space for them to respond to their growth opportunity and health expression innately, which often results in them wanting to be quiet, lie down, eat less, rest and cuddle up to Mum and Dad. Avoid the 'pain' word as it can create a sense of wrongness and urgency in their

experience that fosters fear and being out of control. Their experience is one that is inevitable in life and you have the opportunity to help them shape the amount of stress and fear associated with that experience.

3) Get excited about the opportunity that lies ahead for your child as they move through a health expression. With any health expression, you're alerted to the fact that changes are afoot internally. Creating the opportunity to celebrate those changes allows the child to be comfortable with them. (See Chapter 15: Health Conversations: "Welcome to Our House!")

4) Our house has no medications, homeopathic drops, or natural remedies. Our children have never seen me or their dad taking something to take something away. They don't associate with a 'this for that' scenario. We DO create health expressions and our children see us handling what we have created in a very different way to most households, so we lead by example with congruency in our message.

Our children's perceptions and experiences of sickness is vastly different to many of their peers. They believe in their body's ability to be well and heal as do my husband and I. What they do have that is regular in their life are neurological adjustments by a trained chiropractor—us. All have been adjusted within thirty minutes of their birth and then every week for the whole of their life. We emphasise to our children that they are self-healing, self-regulating and self-regenerating organisms that are constantly adapting to their environment which at times may be challenging but it's always perfect.

What are you pushing?

Ah ha!

* Do you see occasions when you have 'pushed drugs' onto your children?

* How do you want to shape your response to your child's health expression?

* When you or your child next creates a health expression, look for the opportunities that lie ahead because of the changes that are taking place.

CHAPTER 13

The Health Shift: Evolve Your Health or Revolve It!

'Find out what everybody else is doing and run like hell in the opposite direction!'

—— John Ham

When I was growing up during the '70s and '80s the allopathic approach was THE approach to utilise when you wanted to get your 'health' back, or rather to lessen the noise the symptoms were making by taking something to take them away. The indoctrinated system had a stranglehold on parents as they dutifully continued to do what they had always done: go to someone to get something to take something away, done that way because that is the way it has always been done.

Television was new in our town, at least for our family, and the ads shown were targeted at mothers who had most of the responsibility for making the health decisions for their children. Pharmaceutical companies could now place a product ad on TV with a quick few lines about its 'benefits' as well as a visual representation, versus the old radio waves where only the intonation of a commentator's voice could be heard and nothing could be seen. Changes in the quantity of products sold and brand type were noted by marketing experts around the country, and indeed the globe. The TV marketing blitz of drugs was working.

When I was beginning to ask different questions about life and health, my dad shared with me a pearl of wisdom. We were sitting at home in the lounge room and when I finished asking more than likely my tenth question within an hour his head, as quick as a flash, darted from behind the newspaper. Chin lowered and looking over his glasses, he said 'Find out what everybody else is doing and run like hell in the opposite direction!' So when it came time to getting really serious about organising the world's health information into bite-sized pieces so people could understand it, I began looking for where there might be a herd running in the opposite direction.

It wouldn't take long to find one!

In the 1990s it was demonstrated that there was a slow and steady shift occurring in how people were approaching health. No longer were people racing to get the 'fix'; there appeared to be a 'pause' moment and a shift in people's behavior.

During the '90s three significant 'things' happened:

> 1) Our wonderful baby boomers the world over continued to push the boundaries by asking more questions and push the boundaries of 'normal' behaviour;

> 2) The internet started with 24/7 access globally; and

> 3) Information began to be openly shared via people's computers in their own homes.

Information once only allowed for people 'in the know' was now becoming public knowledge. The 'powers that be' were too late in attempting to regulate and censor the information people were able to access—the human element in stories and a sharing of personal truth. Ordinary people were reading the stories of people in Australia, Europe, UK, USA, New Zealand, India, South America and elsewhere. Suddenly the widespread access of information increased people's personal power as they read how people were changing their lives via what was considered unconventional and unscientific ways and 'jumped online' to search 'Dr Google' to investigate their own symptoms and empower themselves with their own decision making. They slowly but surely began making different choices for themselves and their children. People were making the shift; the exodus from the allopathic health approach began.

The allopathic approach—the 'top dog'—had started to crumble ever so slightly. The majority of the world's population still predominately uses the allopathic approach—an outside-in, feeling, food and fitness definition. However, there has been a slight tipping of the scales.

Let's look at it like this …

I imagine you now acknowledge there *are* three health approaches—allopathic, alternative and alternate—each offering the health conscious consumer something unique and each with its place in health because each exists. The question to ask, however, goes back to the health triangle and where you chose to enter that. Knowing about each approach will give you confidence in deciding which approach to use when. Having just read the chapters I'm sure you can see the distinct differences.

For decades there has been one health approach (allopathic, medicine) that wanted to own all of the pie versus dividing the pie evenly into thirds. And like a kid wanting more pie, (ownership over where the people went) it did whatever they could to get more pie (See Chapter 11: Are You a Health Slider?). Others (eg alternate, chiropractic) who had a smaller portion wised up and hung onto their share. Consumers, through books such as this one and my other book *The Vital Truth*,® are now able to understand how the pie is divided and how big pharma cuts their share of it!

To make this point a little clearer …

In the early 1990s a study was done by Dr Eisenberg of Harvard Medical School. He demonstrated for the first time in history there were **more visits to alternative health professionals than there were to all mainstream medical doctors and specialists *combined*.** There were approximately **thirty-eight million more visits to alternative health professionals** than to the medical 'establishment.'

And …

The people using this alternative to health were generally 25 – 49 yrs of age.

Then, in 1997, the same study was repeated with even more stark (if unsurprising) results.

In the US alone there **were 629 million visits to alternative health professionals and only 386 million visits to primary care medical doctors**—nearly twice as many visits and—get this—people were paying out of their own pocket. They paid because they wanted to go. Interestingly when I ask people in an audience when I share this 'piece' of the pie I ask where do they think all the people were going? What was the number one health profession the people were heading towards? Most yell out 'naturopath!'

What Dr Eisenburg found was that people were going to chiropractors—the alternate health approach—the largest regulated and licensed health profession in the world using no drugs or surgery. People en mass began to entertain the idea of staying well and functioning well rather than oscillating around an arbitrary line chasing feelings and symptoms. It simply costs less to function well.

People were asking themselves, 'What is health?'

They began seeing that the alternative approach to health had an answer, and the exodus began. As a result there was a scrambling within the allopathic community as they came to grips with what the study meant to them and the future of health as *they knew it*. In an effort to retain their position, the allopathic profession set out to discredit and shut down individuals—and even whole professions— and at times was successful. Remember from the principle of 'the one and the many' what the 'top dog' position does? They want to own and discredit everything and everyone below them—individuals to organisations to professions—if it will have an impact of their share of the pie and the bottom dollar.

I imagine you could be strung right now between health worlds, wondering if you should jump or not. Or perhaps you want to be over 'there' however you're too scared as to what you might find or see? I offer you this ... start by reading other people's stories to get yourself inspired. You can find 13+ great ones in my book *The Vital Truth*®which is available for immediate download from our Vital Moms website (www.Vitalmoms.com). This book is about creating the initial steps to open your world to seeing health differently, taking charge, having courage and being confident with the decision you make. I know I didn't get to where I am today in my health and in my approach by following the 'conventional' way. I took the time to learn, look and then go see; I decided to stay. **You can always go back *to the way it has always been done*** however I feel with the views I've shared here in this book you're going to find it empowering and inspirational to keep moving forward!

Remember: find out what everybody else is doing and run like hell in the opposite direction!

 Ah ha!

- Find out what everybody else is doing and run like hell in the opposite direction.
- Are your friends approaching health in the same way they always have and nothing seems to be changing? Yes? Than is it time to find some new friends more akin to your new way of thinking? Vital Moms club, www.vitalmoms.com/club, is a great place to start!
- If you watch TV in your house, mute the ads!
- Don't be scared to make a move—go see—there are people to help you.
- Sometimes we worry about what we may lose rather than what we may gain when we decide to do something different.

CHAPTER 14

Lying Lexicon

'The great enemy of the truth is very often not the lie, deliberate, contrived and dishonest, but the myth, persistent, persuasive and unrealistic.'

—— John F. Kennedy

I believe that this chapter and what I have discovered through looking at the language of health will leave you saying 'Wow!' It will also begin to unravel more of the confusion consumers have about health, what it is and where it comes from, simply by looking at the language we use. You will be introduced to the power of language as it relates to health meaning, values and beliefs. If you would like to instigate some changes in your language either in your house, with your children or simply with your own self talk, then make sure you read the 'Lying lexicon' resource, a step-by-step plan to begin incorporating your new words. It's too big to put in here! Details on how to do that are at the end of the chapter.

Let's jump right in …

Seeing we are looking at the lexicon of health, we must briefly revisit each of the health approaches—allopathic, alternative and alternate. These health approaches are both subtly *and* starkly different from each other. In order to change your health approach you have to change your language. It's imperative to know what the differences are between the approaches to be congruent with the one you are choosing. Two of the health approaches are the antithesis of each other in their approach and philosophy (amongst other things) and the other approach, well, it pretty much sits with a mixed understanding of the two health approaches that flank it either side. Understanding the philosophical backgrounds of the three health approaches will begin to show you why we have so much 'consumer confusion' in today's society.

Once we revisit the different health approaches you'll notice fairly quickly whether you are congruent with that health approach or not. It may also become blindingly obvious that you have 'consumer confusion' whereby you engage a 'lying lexicon' within the health approach you use. Umm ... in other words you may find that you are using the language of another health approach when communicating about the health approach you use, which leaves the person you are chatting with absolutely confused and you with an identity health crisis!

Here's the quick review:

ALLOPATHIC e.g. medicine	ALTERNATIVE e.g. everything else!	ALTERNATE e.g. chiropractic
Pathic	Native	Nate
Remaining passive	Offering a choice	In-born
Lucky or unlucky Chance	Lucky or unlucky Chance	Perfect Choice

ALLOPATHIC e.g. medicine	ALTERNATIVE e.g. everything else!	ALTERNATE e.g. chiropractic
Surrender responsibility	Surrender responsibility	Active participant in creating your health
Treatment	Treatment	Adjustment
Fear and 'what if' responses	Fear and 'what if' responses	Trust and change
No intelligence	Inner intelligence	Innate intelligence
Atom smallest component	Atom smallest component	Vibrations, Energy, light (+ and – charge)
Outside-In	Outside-In	Inside-out
Drugs and Surgery	Natural Remedies	Nerve system—master communicator
Diagnosis	Suggestions	Empowering the individual with their own knowing
Need an immediate answer	Time to decide	Decision's yours / It's your body & life
Health = how you **FEEL**	Health = how you **FEEL**	Health = how you **FUNCTION**

I have 'been in' all three of these health approaches at some point in my life: **allopathic, alternative and alternate.** Allopathic when I was very young, alternative in my later teens to mid 20s and since my mid 20s I have chosen to approach my health and life from the alternate approach and have not utilised the other two for either myself or my children. What I have noticed is they all exist, so all are needed, however I feel the scales need some tipping. I respect that all three approaches have distinct differences and philosophical beliefs. I would argue that most people believe there is only one way to approach health and because of that belief they see health as linear; unaware of the choices available. **The approach you use is usually the approach taught to you by your mother, father, teacher, preacher, caregiver, TV, radio, print media and now social media.** In the main, especially in western developed countries, this approach is the allopathic approach. The allopathic approach can come in other guises: modern medicine, mainstream healthcare, the mechanistic approach, or for the sake of simplicity, the 'quick fix', a treatment, or symptomatic relief.

The alternative approach is also referred to as the Complementary and Alternative Medicine or 'CAM' for short as well as natural, integrative, environmental, 'green', allied, esoteric medicine and energy medicine, depending on who is describing it. In short, however, this approach remains mechanistic in its general aim of fixing the body. This is where the largest 'bucket' of health *professions* sit. This approach encapsulates those professions not dispensing pharmaceutical drugs or laboratory-made medications of any kind, but rather 'natural remedies' to assist the body.

The *alternative* approach is deemed just that, by the 'allopathic profession', who see the alternative health approach as 1) unscientific, bordering on hippy, quackery and way out and 2) is exactly what the name implies: an alternative to 'X'. In other words, you'll still get something to take something away, it just won't be a pharmaceutical-grade pill, tablet or medication.

I remember hearing a debate on a US radio station between a professor of Chinese medicine and acupuncture and a medical professor on the validity of the alternative approach. The medical professor was consistently driving home the differences between mainstream medicine (his work) and the alternative approach. Eventually the Chinese medicine professor became quite indignant and reminded the other guest that Chinese medicine was based on a 5,000 year history of both clinical and empirical science, however, western or mainstream medicine had only been around for around seventy-five years! His question was, 'Who is the alternative in this instance?'

There is another crucial point here which contributes to confusion. Many professions who sit in the alternative approach have a desire to be as well known, acknowledged and respected as the allopathic approach. Remember the 'top dog' position? They are the ones seen to have respect and credibility. Well, the alternative professions, over a long period of time (decades) began to adopt similar identities—language, processes, clothing, systems, technology, and philosophy—to that of the allopathic approach in a belief that this will get them to the 'top dog' position; which of course leaves you ... the consumer ... *confused!* Many of these professions struggle within themselves playing what can only be described as the classic game of Twister!

Let's look at it this way ...

I'm sure you have played the game of Twister; most people have. Someone spins the wheel which lands on a colour. You then put a hand (left or right) or a foot (left or right) on the coloured dot that came up when you spun. It's a fun game with the aim being to topple the person; the last person standing wins. Sound familiar?

The more of your body you have on one dot the stronger you are—you're solid and aligned, it's hard to topple you in the game of Twister. However,when you have one hand on the yellow dot, a foot on a blue dot and another foot on a green dot you become unstable, 'a sitting duck' to be toppled at any spin of the wheel. And this is exactly what happens to health professions. The 'top dog' stands firm, anchored, not budging, clear on their beliefs and the direction they are heading. The 'many' attempt to push and shove and grab at anything and everything to be like the 'one'. However they have an unsteady base: spread thin, stretched out, and they topple, get chewed up, displaced, shut down. Game over.

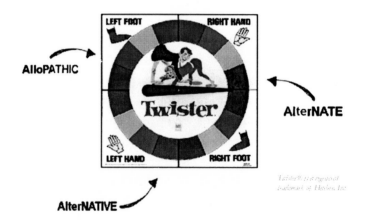

So if a *profession* is confused with the philosophical alignment on which that *profession* was founded than look out! As that profession attempts to morph into something it is not, there is plenty of opportunity to be gobbled up or, at worst, regulated by someone other than itself. Not only does that inherently confuse the professionals within the profession where some want to align with the 'top dog' and others want to stand tall and firm, but it also means the consumer—you—will be confused!

Oh dear.

It's time to stick to what each health profession was founded on rather than mold to another profession's approach. Remember all are needed by virtue of all existing. As I tell my children it's always best to be yourself and beat your own drum.

This is where language becomes such a part of our entrenched cultural thinking and nomenclature.

In understanding the game of Twister and this intense need that professions have to be 'the one' I'm sure you can see how easy it is nowadays for a person to move from the allopathic approach to the alternative. There is safety, it's less threatening, it looks similar to the allopathic approach and they speak a similar language. People are still going to someone to get something to take something away. The mechanistic philosophy that drives the alternative approach is the same as the allopathic approach; even though the *professions* that sit in the alternative approach *are different, the approach is the same.*

The alternate approach expands the understanding of health and the workings of the body. It therefore inherently changes the way health is approached. The allopathic approach and its health language has been successfully ingrained in our culture, permeating our legal, health and political systems. It can be challenging to change and create an alternate congruent health belief and language ... but not impossible, if that is what you would like to do.

Let's take a look now at some common health words and how these words are defined within the allopathic and alternative approaches and what alternate words/language are available.

'Sick'/ 'Sickness' OR 'Health Expression'

When my husband and I decided to have children, I remember thinking about how we would raise them and explain health to them. Of course it would need to be congruent with the way we approached health, which is via the alternate approach. I first acknowledged that I wanted to have a language that would be empowering to use when describing their own or another's health concern or challenge. I see my children as self-healing, self-regenerating and self-regulating human beings who are constantly adapting to their environment. So I wanted words that would be encouraging as opposed to words or statements such as 'you're sick'.

My first word to reframe was 'sickness'. I asked myself what would be an empowering alternate substitute word or phrase. I didn't want our kids to think of themselves as being *sick* but instead think of themselves as expressing health *differently* when those *sick* times arose. So I coined the term **'health expression' to replace 'sickness'**. Our kids use this language with friends and their friend's parents too. At times I see the odd sideways stare accompanied with a wrinkling of the forehead suggesting *'you created a what?'*

But in an alternate approach it makes sense. Using the term **health expression** removes the negative connotation of the word *sickness,* which implies a person is ill which implies that their body has got it wrong, it's suffering—happened to them—when, in fact, the body is attempting to do the best it can given whatever has been created and send the specific messages (symptoms) it wants to alert you to. We have determined over the years that there is a great deal of further discussion and discovery available with our children when we focus on the creation of a health expression. We discuss how well the body is working and how much stronger their bodies will be for the effort it is making in creating a more supportive environment. We ask them where in their lives they feel the health expression will serve the greatest. Remember the 3Ts? Thoughts (emotional), Trauma (physical), and Toxins (chemical). This becomes an opportunity for them to see how their body is working with them and not in spite of them.(See Chapter 15: Welcome to Our House—Health Conversations)

The creation of a health expression has also allowed us to address pain in a very different way to most families. How we perceive pain, which is a central component of the allopathic approach to health, is pivotal to how we then respond to others and of course heal our self. Our children have not anchored an association of victim to their pain, discomfort and/or signs and symptoms; rather they simply allow themselves to have an experience of a health expression. They don't ask us to give them something to take something away, that process is not in their psyche. They do, however, ask for water, a cuddle, or for something to eat, to lie down and of course they often ask if they can get adjusted—not because something is wrong but because everything is right. We adjust our children every week and have done since birth, regardless of what is being expressed.

Many people have asked us, 'What do you do when your child is screaming … or … has a fever … or is in pain … or their ear really hurts and they won't stop crying?'

Our response?

We have not had either of our three kids express *extreme* degrees of health. Some readers might be saying 'Oh, you're lucky.'

My response is **'No, it all goes back to how you are choosing to approach health and educate and explain health to your children.'** Attending to our children's physical, chemical and emotional wellbeing and weekly adjustments means they have not experienced those depths of a health expression that someone else might have experienced. And yes they have had fevers, coughs, runny noses, spots on their bodies, bee stings, sprained ankles, deep cuts, ear aches, deep mucous coughs, sore throats, and skate board, biking, rugby and surfing accidents, like any other child. The difference has simply been in how we have approached health and educated our children regarding that message. Our children, from birth, have been brought up to understand that **health is choice not chance** and everything that is expressed is because they chose to have that experience. A lot can be said for taking a different, alternate approach to health.

If we—and you—are going to raise children in a different approach to health, at least different to the majority of society, then it makes sense to be congruent with the language of the approach chosen.

'Diagnosis'

In the allopathic approach, you remain a passive participant which becomes cemented when you take on board a diagnosis. A diagnosis is important within the allopathic community because it establishes a linear pathway of cause (symptoms) and effect (treatment), even though the cause and effect is defined by your symptoms alone. So really what you are looking for in the allopathic and alternative approach is someone to tell you what you have—a *diagnosis*—so you can get the 'matching thing' to take it away.

However, when you look at the root meaning of the word *diagnosis* you may be surprised with what you read. When you break down the meaning of this word you get to see how words can subtly play with you, creating the health illusion bubble.

In Latin *Di* means 'two' and *agnostic* means 'unknown', or 'don't know'. So really, diagnosis means two [people] who don't know! So why do we diagnose? Umm …

'Treatment'

We see treatment being used consistently within the first two health approaches: allopathic and alternative. It is used loosely without any understanding of its root meaning. Not many people (unless you're a word nerd like me) have taken the time to question the word most commonly used to describe what a person receives when they 'get sick'.

Let's break it down …

In Latin *treat* means 'to deal with' and *ment* means 'mind'. Treatment means *to deal with the mind*. And that is exactly what happens, isn't it? People believe the symptoms are working against them, not for them, and accordingly want them dealt with, taken away and at worst removed. In wanting them dealt with they receive a treatment—that deals with their **mind only**—creating a health illusion that the symptoms (and signs) are no longer there, giving the person a false sense of security that they are healthy again because they feel fine once more.

What a merry-go-round this is!

Before long you will create something else within your body that has you notice the symptoms once more. You yet again jump on the merry-go-round of going to someone, to get something, to take something away … to treat you … to play with your mind. Nothing alters except the treatment of your mind.

Einstein said **'Insanity is doing the same thing over and over again expecting a different result'** and yet people do this when it comes to their health.

The opposite word for treatment in the alternate health approach is the word *adjustment*. This is a word unique to the alternate approach to health. What does it mean? A dictionary definition would give us something like *making a correction*, or *fine tuning something*, but if we take a look at the root meaning of the word we see something more: *ad* means 'move to' *just* means 'centre' and *ment* means 'mind'. Adjustment means *move the mind to centre; to balance.*

An adjustment utilizes three 'things':

    1) a person's internal healing capability;

    2) a person's innate intelligence; and

    3) the nerve system.

All three come together during and post an adjustment to instigate the health changes a person chooses to express. Here the adjustment is looked as the ability of the mind to resume a centre point into balance to once again make different decisions for one's self. Nothing is being treated in this approach. Often people who utilise the alternate approach are found, post an adjustment, saying 'I am not sure what happened, but I am thinking clearer!' … moving the mind back to centre.

When I say 'adjustment,' I'm talking about a specific, slight and purposeful force applied into the body in a precise direction. This opens up communication within the nerve system. The aim is to gently allow the body to move to a natural state of balance and adapt to an ever-changing internal and external environment. To give you an idea of how it works, picture the old TV 'rabbit ears' antennae for a moment. Do you remember a time when your television went all fuzzy? (That's going to depend on how old you are!) Well, what did you do? I imagine you stood up, walked over to the antennae and adjusted the rabbit ears ever so specifically, slightly and purposefully until you received a clearer picture. That is exactly what the alternate approach to health does, e.g. a chiropractor. Adjustments instigate the nerve system to communicate with itself, which in turn allows clearer communication to be expressed throughout the body.

Here's another word ...

'Pharmacy'

Can you see the word within this word? 'Harm' is spelt as clear as day within the word itself.

Meanings within meanings! Interesting.

What about the word **'Try'**?

My dad was a man of little words and a lot of statements and phrases, as you've read. He taught me about the word 'try' in a moment, with his classic look over a newspaper. I was young and asked for some assistance to write a letter for a job I wanted to go for. He said 'Well, you start it and then we can take a look together.'

I was irritated because I really wanted him to write it for me. As I walked off in a huff I said, 'Okay, I'll try.' Down went the paper, his head appeared from behind it and out it came ... another statement: 'There is no such thing as try; you either do it or you don't!'

I learnt that lesson fast! And it's true. Here is a classic example: try and stand up? There is no 'try,' you either do it or you don't! And you're not going to 'try' and create health—you either will or you won't. Trying is closely aligned to an illusion. You create a false feeling of 'doing something' when really you're either doing it or you're not.

I remember many a time growing up using the word 'can't'. Again I received a mighty lexicon lesson! I only wish I saved all the 'statements' I'd call it *John Ham's little book of sayings*. This one came back at me loud and clear, and interestingly I hear myself saying it to my kids who know it really well! As soon as I'd say 'I can't' he would reply with 'Three-quarters of that word, Sarah, says *can*. What you're really saying is that you won't.'

'Damn!' I used to say to myself. 'You are too smart!' And yet again is true.

I've listed below some statements commonly associated with each of the health approaches:

Allopathic & Alternative Language	Alternate Language
Fear: 'What if I don't take this?'	Trust: 'I trust all in my world is perfect.'
Passive: 'They told me I had to.'	Active: 'I'll decide if I will ...'
Surrender: 'I have to take 'x, y, z.'	Accountability: 'I'm going to ...'
Unlucky: 'It just happened to me.'	Choice: 'I created ...'
Victim: 'I didn't do anything; it just happened.'	Responsible: 'I chose to ...'
'He's got a... / She caught a...' / 'I have a...'	'He / She created a ...'
'I think so but I'm not sure.'	'I know ...'
'I can't...'	'I can ...'

I want you to notice here how closely the words are aligned to the *remaining passive participant role* people play when they use the allopathic and alternative approach. It is fascinating to see how language plays such a hefty role in cementing beliefs about health and the body's ability, and either empowering you or disempowering you.

Here are some other words which keep you on the merry-go-round:

Sick: 'to chase'

Ill: 'sick'

Ill-u-sion—ill = 'sick', u = 'u', ion = 'condition of' there for illusion = condition of [keeping] you sick!

Ah ha!

- What language are you reinforcing as you learn about health and teach that to your children?

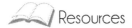 Resources

'Lying lexicon'
<u>www.VitalMoms.com/healthillusion</u>

CHAPTER 15

Health Conversations: 'Welcome to Our House!'

'The most influential of all educational factors is the conversation in a child's home.'

—— William Temple

Welcome to our house! I'm going to share a few typical conversations that Randall and I have had with our children to demonstrate the 'pathway' we took in having our kids reach a conclusion for themselves, with our guidance. There are numerous stories I could share here spanning years across three children. However I have chosen just a few to get you started in your house.

I knew while I was pregnant with our first and sitting firmly in this alternate approach to health that it would make sense to be congruent with the approach my husband and I had chose to 'be in'. To do that I had to have a language specific to that approach otherwise I was simply confusing them—playing Twister! In order for me to do that I made a commitment prior to our eldest's birth to 'pause', to respond rather than react, to be me and to always share my truth. After all, they had chosen me to be their mother. As such I invented my own words (e.g. health expression Vs sickness) and decided I wouldn't read any how-to parenting books— that indeed if I did I would be 'checking at the door' part of who I am every time I went to have a conversation or an experience with them. I didn't want that. So I decided that if I'm going to 'show up' as their parent then they are going to get all of me—the good, the bad and the ugly as the saying goes, the part that makes mistakes and the part that gets it right—they get it all.

As I'm navigating the parent path I see my role as a mum as giving each of my children wings. You'll notice that during my conversations with them I am attempting to place another bow in their quiver of life, to be drawn upon as needed by them when they're ready. You'll read conversations about health and life, because I see the alternate approach to health as a 'way of life' philosophy too.

Enjoy the conversations.

Our youngest: 'the audition'

My husband asked the kids if they would like to audition for 'The Sound of Music' musical coming to town. They all jumped with excitement at the opportunity to display their talent. However as the time got closer we noticed anxiety, fear and 'what ifs' starting to surface. At dinner one night we all went around the table sharing the emotions being felt of a day yet to come. My husband and I helped each of the kids reach their own conclusions about what they were feeling.

I shared at the table that night some wisdom about building a wall.

'When you build a wall (e.g. get the part) you can either become overwhelmed at the thought of building a wall (getting a part) and therefore be paralyzed by the thought OR you can say to yourself 'I'm going to lay a brick, one brick, as best as I can, as perfectly as I can in the moment to help build my wall'; doing so consistently enough will build your wall.'

So we gave the wall a name and called it the 'Wall of Experience'.

After I'd finished and they had contemplated what I had shared, our middle boy came to us and after much contemplation (sleep) he said 'Mum, I really am the rugby boy. This isn't my thing.'

I asked him what he would like to do it. He said 'I would prefer not to audition.'

'Okay,' I said.

My eldest and youngest decided to 'give it ago.'

The day arrived. I made them a huge yummy home-cooked, organic breakfast, adjusted them and then off we went to the venue—lunch packed, numbers pinned onto their shirts and the 'wall of experience' etched in their minds. You could tell they were nervous when we arrived but they quickly made friends with other kids in the queue, switching their minds to other things. Slowly each character group was called out and taken into the massive 2,000 seat theatre—on their own, no parents allowed.

While the kids were auditioning I had the opportunity to share with other parents. Most were concerned for their child and how they would handle the disappointment if they didn't get in. They were asking me questions about how to comfort their child—I must have looked like someone who had the answer! I shared with them about experiences versus expectations. That placing an expectation on themselves will inherently create a disappointed child if they didn't get a part. I shared what I had shared with our children: that life is a series of experiences and they have an opportunity from birth to death to create a 'wall of experience' and that 'laying a brick' was but one part of creating the wall. Each brick, for instance, represents their audition experience and eventually with enough bricks laid (experience had) they will have their wall (their moment, their part).

Parents were grateful for the conversation. When the children come out of the theatre and told they had not got a part most melted, crying in their mothers' arms. As my eldest and youngest came out separately from their audition they each mentioned the 'wall of experience'. Our eldest said 'that was an experience, Mum; I've laid that brick ... I'll stick to swimming!' Our youngest, well, she came bounding out towards me, big smile on her face and hugging me said 'Mummy, Mummy, I didn't get in but I laid a brick!' She wants to do it again. I was excited for each of them and how they handled their experience.

We bundled up our belongings, repacked the back packs and headed out the theatre door. As we were walking out I overheard a mum saying to her child 'you've laid a brick.' I smiled at the thought of helping a family, a child, have a different experience.

Our middle boy: 'full circle'

Rui is hilarious, the cheeky one and always has us in stitches in a split second. He is delightful to be around with his gung-ho, fast paced wit! He also has a serious side to him; tender and kind.

We were driving to our regular café, just the two of us, heading out for some time together and some lunch. He was sitting in the front and chatting away. I'd hear a muffled question being asked and reply 'What was that'? 'Say that again?' 'I can't hear you. What did you say?' The radio wasn't on so I knew I couldn't blame it on the music being too loud to hear him. He then shouted in frustration '*Mum* ... are you listening to me?' As I jumped a little I replied, 'Actually, no I wasn't'

'Well, I was telling you about what happened at rugby training.'

I said 'My head's preoccupied, I'm creating a health expression. What did you want to say?'

He turned to me, tapped me on my arm and said 'Good job, Mum health expression. Growth opportunity. So what's it about: physical, chemical or emotional?' Interestingly, I heard him—and roared with laughter! He continued 'Perhaps we can take some time over lunch, Mum, to find out what it is.'

Priceless. Children are great mirrors and teachers when we take the time to listen and learn from them as well. Indeed, that is exactly what we did!

Our eldest boy: 'possibility'

Anam has been swimming since 2012. However, because we live on an island he only gets to swim for four months of the year, three times a week for an hour at a time. The rest of the year he doesn't swim at all as there is no indoor or warm pool on the island.

This was his second year of competitive swimming. He is a wonderful swimmer, graceful to watch and has his heart set on competing for a country—he has a choice. As part of his home education I suggested he write his times down in a book. He thought that would be a good idea too and set about ruling up a small exercise book which wasn't being used. He wrote his times down and worked on beating his personal best times each week. He came to me one day and asked if we could look up the fastest times in his age group. So we sat at the computer and began the journey into finding out what they were. As we looked and he wrote down the times he noticed in one of his strokes there was a twelve second difference. I noticed his shoulders began to slump and his facial expression reflect the thought of 'Can I beat that?'

On one site there was a video which I clicked on. It was of a young girl who was an outstanding swimmer at her club. The video covered her training schedule which was ten sessions a week for up to two hours at a time— starkly different to what our son does. The interviewer asked this young girl what her favourite meal was and she mentioned a well-known fast food chain. I was horrified. Anam was also wondering why people can eat junk and still perform well. He left the room. After closing the computer and heading to the dinner table I wondered how I could turn what we just saw, heard and read into a conversation where he can reshape for himself what that time difference actually meant.

While we were eating dinner I asked Anam what he thought about the time difference. He shrugged, clearly feeling rather despondent with how it could be changed. I shared with him that perhaps he wasn't twelve seconds slower, but rather he had available to him twelve seconds of possibility. His eyes darted up from his plate to look at me, his ears pricking up a little too.

'Where are your twelve seconds of possibility?'

He paused and said 'I get adjusted every week', to which I replied, 'How many seconds is that worth to you?'

He said 'Three seconds.'

I said 'What else?'

'I eat homemade and organic food?'

'Great! How many seconds is that worth to you?'

'Three seconds.' 'Great! What else?'

'I could get a coach who would work on my technique.'

'How many seconds is that worth to you?'

'Five seconds.'

'Great! What else?' I asked.

'You and Dad help me a lot with my mental thoughts and belief in myself.'

'How many seconds is that worth to you?'

'Three seconds,' he said.

'How many seconds are you at now?'

He added them up and said 'Fourteen seconds.'

'Are you ahead?' I asked.

'Yes.'

'By how much?'

'Two seconds!'

I then shared with them all that we could have looked at our eldest being twelve seconds slower and ended the conversation with 'Well, if you want it bad enough, train harder and get fitter.' However, that is not how we chose to frame this experience because in reality that is not true.

We chose to share the truth and the truth is that the time difference is equivalent to twelve seconds of possibility. Sport, I said, is about the whole self—it isn't about one aspect of you—the fast one or the coordinated one or the fit one. It is about ALL of you and the choices you make while training for what you want. The 'whole of you' is the important part; all aspects present all aspects of oneself needed.

I summed up our conversation by saying we all have possibility. What we do with that possibility makes all the difference to our own success. It's the one who acknowledges the differences and believes they truly have 'x' seconds of possibility that enables their inner champion to shine.

Our youngest girl: 'Ow'

We have always taught out children about the 3Ts: thoughts (emotional), trauma (physical) and toxins (chemical) from a very young age. I didn't have special language in communicating with them—a baby language—I only chose to use the English language and speak to them as I would to any other person I was speaking to. I trusted that our children were born with intelligence and as such their neurological filters would be able to understand what I was communicating—verbally, visually and by my actions and their observations of those actions.

Anais' was a breech birth at home and out of all three of our children she is the one to create ear challenges. I adjust her and tuck her into bed with me. Hugging her, I begin to ask her questions about her ear. I asked her, in a more recent example, what's going on. At first sure wasn't sure and I reassured her that she did know. I continued to ask the same question, 'What's going on?' She said 'I created a health expression.'

'I can see that. What's it about?

She paused and said 'I don't know.'

I confidently said, 'Yes you do. Is it physical, chemical or emotional?'

'Chemical.'

'Health expression, chemical body. What's going on there?'

'I ate too much of something.'

'What was the something you ate too much of?'

'Honey,' she said. 'I ate too much honey.' She began to cry a little as she settled into bed. I lay with her all tucked in; hugging her. She said 'Mummy, will you hold my ear?' I said yes. Anais started to go 'ow' as she told me where to pull on her ear lobe. I stopped when I heard her say 'Just there, Mummy.'

As she lay saying 'ow' I said 'Let's together, after every 'ow' say 'wow'.'

Until she drifted off to sleep that night that's exactly what we did … 'ow'… 'wow'. I spoke about her inner guidance, her innate intelligence, the opportunity and possibility about to unfold for her in the days to come.

Following any health expression created by our children we have always asked in what way do they feel the health expression will benefit them. I explain natural immunity is built within 7-14 days and hence post a heath expression at approximately ten days there will be a shift—perhaps it is food, dexterity, strength, friends, clothing choice, height and so forth. The possibilities are endless. As a parent I have great delight in noticing the changes and celebrating these changes with them.

Our middle boy: 'I like what they're doing'

For many years Rui has expressed his health challenges through his skin, predominantly rashes and sores. At the time of this conversation we didn't consume wheat but did have other grains. He would sometimes go to the bakery next door to our practice and buy himself something, even though it was not something we espoused. He also would be given white bread, plastic cheese and cordials and the like at friend's houses. I had, of course, no control over this other than letting the parents know that his body reacts to those types of foods and trust that they would support his body by not feeding him processed 'food' items.

His body was beginning to respond in a magnified way.

At every step along the journey I asked him to notice the changes his body was demonstrating. He was able to see where it was affecting him most—his lips, neck and his lower back—inflammation, redness, and unhealed sores. All present to alert him to something had to change. It got to a stage where I said 'Perhaps it would be good if you stopped going to your friend's house if you are not being nutritionally supported or responsible when you go there. If not, I can make you snacks to take or you can "fill up" before you go. What do you want to do?'

He opted to stop going for awhile.

During this time when Rui's body was expressing his health challenge I spoke about the organ predominately associated with the lips and the lower back area—the bowels. Explaining that the bowels have a series of referral points within the body so that you can 'see' that something needs to be changed according to that organ. 'Something,' (we do not label) I said 'is inside and wants to get out so let's understand your body and work with it to help whatever that is do what it needs to do.' He agreed. I explained that his body wasn't working against him, conspiring in some way to make his life miserable but rather his innate intelligence chose the wisest and fastest route for him to get whatever was in out; he chose his skin.

One Sunday morning I was in my office doing some work while my husband was making the kids breakfast as he does every Sunday. There was a knock on the door and a little head peeked in. It was Rui.

'Morning, Mum, can I speak to you for a moment?'

'Sure darling what would you like to talk about?'

'Well I've been thinking about my lips, neck and my lower back.'

'What have you been thinking?'

'Well I think there is something in what those Paleo people do.'

'What do they do?'

'They don't eat wheat.'

'How is that significant to you?'

'I think I need to stop eating wheat?'

'Do you think or do you know?' I said

'I know, Mum. I need to stop eating wheat'

'Do you need to or do you want to?'

'I want to mum,' he said.

'So what would you like to do and how can I support you in that decision?'

'I'd like you to read more about Paleo and do it with me.'

'Okay,' I said.'We will read together and I'll do it with you.'

His body changed rapidly … within weeks. What was wonderful was noticing his own sense of empowerment over what he had created and the understanding of the dynamic body he chose to inhabit. It was Rui who made the decision to change. Upon making the decision he decided to tell everyone he was 'going paleo,' a sign of the commitment he was making to himself. A new world opened to him that wasn't previously open as people, strangers began sharing their 'paleo story' with him. He felt validated in his choice to change.

Rui became a leader in our house *the day he decided* to do something different; to go paleo—everyone followed.

Our eldest: skate ramp

Prior to moving from the Sunshine Coast in QLD, Australia to New Zealand Anam had created a health expression. I could hear him writhing on his bed one night and said to my husband, 'I'm going to check on Anam.' So up I walked to his room, and sure enough he was writhing around his bed, moaning and half asleep. I knelt down beside him, much like my dad had done with me at the age of seven, and placed my hand knowingly and firmly on his forearm, assuring him that someone was present to his needs.

I said 'Anam, it's Mummy. What's going on?

'I don't know, I don't know,' was his response.

'Yes you do. What's going on?'

'I don't know, I don't know,' was his response again.

'Yes you do. What's going on?'

'Well, clearly I created a health expression.'

'Great! What is the health expression about?'

'I don't know, I don't know.'

'Yes you do. Is it physical, chemical or emotional?'

He paused. 'Physical.'

I began celebrating with him. 'Great! Health expression, physical body. What is the physical about?'

'I don't know.'

'Yes you do. What is the physical about?'

'Well you know the skate park you take us to?'

'Yes.'

'Well, the middle ramp I can't get down.'

'Yes.'

'I think I will grow in my strength and will get down the ramp.'

'Do you THINK or do you KNOW?'

Anam answered, 'I know I will get down the ramp.'

'Great! Health expression, physical body, grow in strength, and get down the ramp. Awesome!' I adjusted him, tucked him in, kissed him good night and off he went to sleep.

Two days later he was down the ramp.

Now that could have been a very different picture in a household that espouses a different approach. Remember that the quality of your life is based on the quality of your questions, and people who utilise this alternate approach respond to trust. I empowered Anam with different questions and my conversation with him came from a place of absolutely knowing that he had the answers inside of him, that he is an intelligent being and has the ability to heal himself.

After all, the only doctor is the one inside of you. I adjusted him, not because something was wrong with his body, but rather because everything was right with his body; knowing full well that a body that can communicate with itself can heal itself.

Our youngest girl: 'agreements and responsibility'

On a morning run with my youngest, we started on an undulating six kilometre track (3.72 miles). Anais is used to it, runs it well and never complains. She agreed to run it with me the night before. She got her clothes out all ready on the bed to put on as soon as she woke. Morning appeared, we got dressed and off we went driving to the overland track. Halfway through she said she was hot, and hot it was—a lovely summer day. So I took a moment to find a wonderful shaded spot on the track with a fabulous view out over the ocean and we sat together and chatted. It didn't matter to me how long the conversation took; what was more important was the opportunity within the circumstance for a life lesson.

I spoke about agreements and responsibility, mentioning that she agreed to come on the run with me knowing full well what was in front of her, the path she was to take and the challenge it would serve. In taking the step forward to participate Anais was accepting the responsibility that went with that decision.

I paused and then painted a picture of her future life, mentioning there will be moments when she will step forward fully aware of what's to come and that there will be challenges in doing so. The question I asked her was 'What can you ask yourself so that in the future you are sure you want to do something? Because,when you step forward, you make a commitment to yourself and those around you.'

Her response? 'Make sure with *my heart* it is something I want to do and not because others want me to do it.'

'Perfect' I said. We hugged each other for what seemed like an eternity and then off she set again with a lightness in her step, having been listened to, heard and empowered.

Sometimes, that's all it takes to have a BIG impact on a child's life ... isn't it?

Ah ha!

- What do you find yourself saying to your children when they are 'sick'?

- Are you trusting that you and your children have all that is required to express health?

- Do you find yourself playing Twister? In other words, intellectually following the alternate health approach and then when a health expression is created, reverting to the approach used by the majority of society, the allopathic approach?

- What steps can you take to hold the alternate health approach in the face of a health expression?

CHAPTER 16

Seven-Year Rotations

'Still round the corner there may wait a new road or a secret gate.'
— JRR Tolkien

DD Palmer, the founder of the chiropractic profession, coined the term 'The 3Ts'. He was referring to Thoughts, Trauma and Toxins. I believe there is additional meaning behind DD's initial finding than he first indicated when he first described the stressors that act on us, interfering with our nerve communication thereby contributing to our signs and symptoms.

Here's what I offer in addition to his discovery ...

During my days training to be a teacher I read about Waldorf Steiner philosophy and I'd studied pedagogics. My husband had done a stint at a Waldorf school in Melbourne so we were aware of its teaching practices and development philosophy. Their philosophy references the 'physical child' throughout the first seven years of life and I completely agree. I've noticed incredible changes with my own children as they have grown through this 0-7 year cycle.

I remember some time ago before nodding off to sleep I asked a simple question 'What comes next ... after the physical body?' I drifted off with an open and curious mind and woke in what seemed like minutes later. I sat upright, reached for my paper and pen, switched on my bedside table light and began writing down everything being said over and over again in my head. When I stopped writing, I immediately drifted back to sleep to awake in the morning with a few 'Ah ha' moments!

I had written that night about three 'cycles'—physical, chemical and emotional. I used to wonder why they, *physical, chemical and emotional*, ran off my tongue so well *in that order* until I noticed that indeed there was an order. I've always imagined the physical, chemical and emotional selves like the points of a triangle—there's that triangle again! And as we journey through the course of life the triangle rotates so a different aspect of our self is pointing forward. The other two are still present, quietly providing input in the back ground ... doing their 'thing' until it is their time to shine.

Every seven years the triangle rotates one 'click' ... transitioning from one to another. I feel you'll enjoy reading what I wrote that night I went to bed and asked 'what comes next?' and you may even crack a smile at the logic behind it. After looking at what I wrote the next question I asked was 'What signifies these changes?' As a mum sitting in the alternate approach to health I looked to the body and life for those answers. I certainly wasn't disappointed. Here's what I wrote:

0-7: physical = growth and neuronal development.

7-14: chemical = puberty.

14-21: emotional = *de*pendence vs *inde*pendence tussle.

21-28: physical = back to the gym to get buffed and shined to go get a mate.

28-35: chemical = reproduction … 'my clock is running out of time'; a fallacy in itself.

35-42: emotional = midlife crises.

42-49: physical = body loosing shape need to head back to the gym to get fit and loose the baby flab.

49-56: chemical = menopause and manopause.

56-63: emotional = retirement where to now, have I lived and done what I wanted to do.

63-70: physical = need to keep moving or 'old age' will set in.

70-77: chemical = old age sets in.

77-84: emotional = *inde*pendent vs *de*pendant tussle, house or retirement home.

84-91: physical = transition to death.

There are many examples I can use to demonstrate each of these stages, however I feel that would all form a book in itself and cover a day of speaking! However for the purpose of making a significant point I would like to choose the first transition a child goes through between 0-7 and 7-14 years and what it signifies is taking place, in the hope that you too will see how remarkable the body truly is.

Here we go …

Lets say your child has hit the all important transition age, a time of great celebration as the body undertakes it's first 'click' of rotation and begins to establish a different set of challenges. A knowing that this transition is underway is the significance of a wobbly (wibbly as our kids called it) tooth! At the age of 6.5 years to 7.5 years children are beginning to lose their baby teeth. Prior to these changes the adult tooth undertakes a tremendous amount of scissoring—up and down—as it begins to slowly but purposefully push its way up and push the baby tooth out. This is the same scissoring action used when a baby tooth is scissoring up and down and pushing through for the first time. As the teeth begin their scissoring action, generally over the months prior there are changes in the cranium. The teeth coming through are bigger and require more space. As the whole cranium expands for the new 'bigger' teeth to fit there are subtle changes in the pituitary gland, the master hormone gland of the body which, of course, instigates the beginning of the next stage—chemicals and puberty. That is a body that knows what it is doing. One 'click' of the triangle and your child is now being 'driven' by another aspect of themselves: their chemical body. Remember, the physical and the emotional are present, however they quietly work together in the background.

This is an important time to make sure your child has a balanced nerve system. This is because your child's cranium (and your own) houses the brain and coming off of the brain is the spinal cord and together they form the central nerve system which is of utmost importance for the child's future growth, development and expression of health. As the cranium makes room for the adult teeth to settle in to their newfound home it too marks a significant transition in how the child sees and interacts with their world. The child subtly begins to seek more of an understanding about the 'self'. Their mind slowly but surely becomes more abstract, seeing themselves for the first time as separate to others. Caution begins to be demonstrated and fear can start to limit certain behaviour. You will notice children sitting for longer periods of time; more pensive in thought. What a well guided body! We found with our children that they began to ask 'how' questions as opposed to 'why' questions. We had questions asked about how rain forms, how did the plants get here, how do the trees grow, how did humans develop as well as many other wonderful 'how' questions. These were purposefully thought out questions; fascinating to witness. You could almost see the cognitive wheels going round in their head!

As each of our children has transitioned into their adult teeth we have also observed changes in their gait (walk). There is a direct relationship between the cranium, the hips, knees, ankles and gait. Changes in the cranium will lead to changes in posture and therefore how a child walks. Ankles become unstable and the hips 'lock' in an attempt to give the body support and stability. We noticed both our boys altered the way they ran when they entered in the 7-9 year age range. Once great runners they, almost overnight, became labored in running style. It was really interesting to observe. However, more importantly, we had them note their changes so they could be empowered by its progress.

I feel as children transition from the 0-7 year age group to the 7-14 year age group we need to pause and celebrate. So many wonderful changes are occurring that if we don't stop to 'see' and observe them we miss it in a timeframe that feels as quick as missing that first step. This is such an important age as their teeth set the stage for future cellular, tissue and organ health. To support your child's changes it's wise to choose the health approach you are aligned to, sit comfortably in it and find health advocates who also 'sit there' to support you in the choices you are making for your children … *in a natural way.*

Resources

'The significance of the wibbly tooth'
www.VitalMoms.com/healthillusion

CHAPTER 17

The Ups and Downs of Pregnancy and Birth

'When you change the way you view birth, the way you birth will change.'
— Marie Mongan

When I was pregnant with our twins, four wonderful Amish trained midwives came into our life. They were beautiful, incredible women who, at the time, had been in the presence of approximately 2,000 birthing women, amongst which were twenty-five sets of twins and there had been only one third stage (birth of the placenta) emergency. All live births. A testament to these Amish trained women *who trust, immerse and ingrain themselves in a belief that a women's body is designed to give birth.* There has not been a 'bad' birth in their books—these are certainly few and far between. What conventional medicine and birthing routines would see as a danger or a disaster brewing, they see as no big deal. They just handle it and get on with letting the woman have the birth experience.

They held meetings at their place once a month to bring birthing mothers and fathers together and to talk about fears, apprehensions and solidify the journey each of us was about to undertake. There were six couples there the day we first went. The topic? 'Our fears'. We sat in a circle on the floor, getting to know each other and sharing lunch. Each person took their turn to say what they wanted to: pain, pressure, ending up in a hospital, disfigured … you name it, there was the full gamut of concerns. Than it was my time to share … 'My greatest fear is that my body doesn't know how to birth'. When I think of what I said then and what I know now, there is a gigantic valley in the middle. However, in my first pregnancy it was very real; uncharted waters with no navigation system, sailing to a destination I knew nothing about.

My fears came to fruition. In March 2001 I created a miscarriage with our twins at fourteen weeks. I didn't know it was twins while I was pregnant because, like the Amish, we did not take part in the medicalisation of the birth journey. No medical doctor, no ultrasounds, no dopplers, no dilation checks … zip, zero, naught, nothing … except for me and my baby—my babies. It was about 10:00 pm and I was at home with my husband, comfortable and quiet. I held the belief that my body didn't know how to birth a baby *naturally* … vaginally, right up until the contractions escalated and my breathing became deeper.

I was raised to be responsible for life's experiences. I acknowledge that this experience didn't happen to me and it wasn't beyond my control, but rather there were circumstances that gently guided the loss and I take full responsibility for the part I played and the part our twins played as intelligent beings—together, perfect. I created this experience for just that: an experience which taught me that indeed my body *does* have everything it requires to birth.

My greatest lesson was one of trust. I didn't race off to have a Dilate and Curate or D&C as they are called, where the surgeon scraps the inside of the uterus wall to make sure everything passed. That went against what I believe about the body and its innate knowing of what to do every time, all the time. I trusted.

Over the next few months, I felt challenged with my hormones. My progesterone had plummeted post-birth, and I was angry, confused, and trapped—feelings I hadn't experienced at this intensity before. Randall noticed the difference in me and decided to take me away to a small town called Galena to a beautiful bed & breakfast, where I could escape the phone and the knocks on the door. Much to my surprise, I took with me some beautiful watercolor paints and a deck of self-healing cards. I wanted to draw, paint, and communicate with our children. During our stay, I was reminded of the birth by each blood clot that still passed through my body, although they were much less frequent. I sat at the window looking out over a field. The weather was cold, and Randall lit the fire. I pulled three cards, one for me and one for each of our children. I asked what I needed to know.

My card said:

'All is well in my world: everything is working out for my highest good. Out of this situation only good will come. I am safe.'

Then I pulled two cards—ironically one was male and one was female. The male card said:

'Life is simple and easy; all that I need to know at any given moment is revealed to me. I trust myself and I trust in life. All is well.'

The female card read:

'I am beautiful, and everybody loves me. I radiate acceptance, and I am deeply loved by others. Love surrounds me and protects me'.

I looked at these cards with an uncanny feeling. At this point, I understood two pertinent epiphanies. One, that nothing is ever missing in our life. We have everything we need; however it just might be in a form we have not yet recognised or experienced. Second, the world exists in balance. Here I am holding our two children: one a male and one a female, having just experienced birth and death with them, the perfect balance. Both of them were teaching me to trust. I went on to sketch the information I received. Upon completion of the drawing and painting, I realized that we indeed hadn't lost our children. I saw that they were in fact still with us. They were now a beautiful painting, which would hang brightly in each of our children's rooms in the years to come. The day after I finished painting, and experienced those epiphanies, the blood flow stopped. No longer did I need to experience the loss. I had our children with us; they were now in a picture form.

Over the next eighteen months, I shared the story of my newfound trust in the body with hundreds of students and people who were eager to hear and learn about the wisdom of the body and philosophy I lived by. In each audience, listeners responded with gratitude that I gave a voice to the innate understanding of the body, which knows what to do every time, all the time. Repeatedly, people would come up to me afterward to share with me the current form of their baby. I lived in awe of the power of the truth I learned to share and felt humbled at the joy people experienced. When the audience realized this universal truth, they experienced a huge relief and an understanding that nothing is ever missing; it just changes form. I was privileged to see listeners able to reconnect with their own little ones, and to recognize the gift that had brought them to this point in their life.

The death and birth of our twins enabled me to awaken the trust inside, to be humbled by the sheer genius of the body we live in. Their death and birth enabled me to ask different questions and to be awakened to new answers. Their death and birth were pivotal in bringing me to where I am today. My life was to be changed forever. My fear might not seem so grand now, after three home birthed children, the last of which was a breech, but after decades of working with women through adjustments both physically, chemically and emotionally I have found this fear in many of their lives. For me the fear was wondering if, in fact, I could birth. 'Could I really do it?' was a question I used to ask myself. I soon came to realise I didn't trust in my body—not myself, not my mind—but my body's ability to birth. Fear and trust became the grappling emotions of my first pregnancy. Our miscarriage, our twins, gave me the firsthand experience of a home birth, the firsthand experience of trust, the firsthand experience of my body's innate design and knowing. I realise the gift the twins gave me was the experience of birth.

. . . .

Anam's birth

August 2001, a few months after the miscarriage of our twins, I was pregnant again. This time there was a different energy, a gleeful pep and excitement in my step. May 2002 would be the month more than likely our 'little one' would be born. We wanted another home birth experience, albeit this one would have a different outcome. We went back to our Amish midwives and asked them to be present at this birth. 'Yes, of course!' was their response. As my pregnancy progressed I heard whispers dotted over the months giving me snippets of information about the birth ... *a Saturday ... eight hours*

... 4:00 pm ... daytime ... lounge room floor ... raining ... stormy ... I trusted, listened and made a mental note.

Isn't it true that when you're pregnant you get a whole lot of unsolicited information pouring your way? When I was pregnant with my eldest I found myself listening to a lady in the aisle of our local Hy-Vee supermarket in the USA, rambling on to me about pain, discomfort and drugs. Her last comment to me as she paid for her groceries was *when it all slows down honey ... take the drugs!* I thought to myself, why is it people feel compelled to share their birth story, good or bad, with you when you are pregnant? I decided that day in the Hy-Vee checkout aisle to surround myself with white light, nod politely and say to myself 'that's your journey, not mine.' As I see it, everybody's journey is different—experiences, birth option, thought processes, trauma, fear, structural integrity and nerve system disturbance, amongst many other factors.

Our eldest's birth was a physical one. We were selling our house, packing boxes, moving countries, and graduating to embark on a new career. My husband was adjusting me and I was receiving adjustments from a chiropractor at the college. We did a neuro-emotional adjustment, asking a series of questions and one of the questions I asked was 'Am I carrying twins?' It returned a positive result. 'Twins, wow!' I was excited. Perhaps they are coming back, I would wonder. We started looking for names and came up with 'Anam Cara' based on the book by John O'Donahue meaning 'soul friends' if one was a boy and one was a girl.

On the morning of May 11ᵗʰ 2002 I awoke at 8:00 am and declared to my husband 'This baby will be born today by 4:00 pm!' Interesting I didn't say 'these' babies; intuitively I felt it was one even though I loved the idea of birthing and parenting twins. Randall filled up the birthing pool we'd hired which sat in the lounge room and I lay in bed, breathing through the mild contractions. I eventually got up to walk the length of our home—up and down, up and down—noting to myself that it was a Saturday.

Everything was 'set' according to Randall ... towels, water, ice, and a Swiss exercise ball which I would sit on during the first stage contractions. As the morning progressed I kept asking Randall what time it was, aware of my 4:00 pm birth declaration! The clouds were rolling in and the light outside started to get dark. The contractions came on in earnest just after midday as the midwives arrived. I drew a sense of 'I can do this' when they walked in. They didn't say anything, they seamlessly slipped in and sat at my feet, whispering to me on occasion. Two were by my feet, one was transcribing by hand everything I said and the other was attending to food and the spa should we require it. As it came to transition and time to enter the second stage—pushing—I stood up and turned around to face my husband. My arms went around his neck, my feet touched each of the midwives and I began pushing—deep breaths. I drew on the intense focus I learnt from my sporting days, no screaming, deep breathing, I trusted. As the pushing eased I looked at my watch and heard the rain and storm hit. I felt cocooned in our home, surrounded with support. After thirteen pushes our eldest graced our presence: 8 hours and 53 minutes, at 4:30 pm. Even though there was only one, we still loved the name Anam meaning 'soul' and so that is what we named him.

Rui's birth

What a ride it was in my second pregnancy. This baby, I felt, was going to be bigger. I noticed the changes in my eating compared to Anam who was tiny, a small 6 lbs 7 oz. I just knew there was something different about this baby. I was working while I was pregnant up until the last two months. I stopped early because I kept having 'false alarms'. Like Anam's pregnancy I was given little whispers. I kept getting the numbers *3, 5 and 8 ... morning ... Saturday ... lounge room ... on own*. Again I trusted, listened and made a mental note.

We were living back in Australia by this time, in QLD. I knew I wasn't going to birth in a hospital nor a birthing suite, home was always where my heart was. I was looking, however, for the equivalent of our Amish midwives I had with Anam. Time was on my side; I had nine months to find the person. Eventually she came into our life via word of mouth, careful not to hand out the details to just anyone as, like the Amish, she worked outside 'the system'—working quietly in the background. I connected with her immediately, however each time she popped in for a cuppa and then left I saw the vision of the birth and she wasn't in the picture. My husband asked a colleague to come around and be present with us and adjust us before and when the birth was in process. He agreed to be that person. Both myself and my husband like someone else to be present to adjust me so he can be the dad and enjoy the moment, knowing he is taken care of as well. And based on my upright arms around his neck as my preferred birth position, we wanted to have someone else there to assist down there!

I went to bed on 29th October, 2004 and was awoken at 3:00 am with contractions that were coming on fairly fast. I softly nudged Randall and quietly said 'this is it.' He jumped out of bed and started to prepare the lounge room: our little blue box, Swiss ball, ice blocks, towels. Randall went outside to the fence and called for Annie, our next door neighbor, who was on 'Anam watch.' I got up not long after Randall, he adjusted me and I began walking the length of the house, similar to what I had done with Anam. I felt everything slowing down and ask Randall to call our colleague and have him come around. It seemed hours until he arrived. I asked to be adjusted immediately and requested a neuro-emotional adjustment; I knew the slowing was nothing to do with the baby and everything to do with me. It was my emotions halting the birth progressing. I was navigating new territory, unsure if I could parent two. Would I have enough to go around? Was it going to be a boy or a girl? Could I continue to work with two children?

Questions, questions ....

Immediately after the adjustment I began my 'on cue' transition sign of deep gagging and vomiting—which helps to dilate and expand the cervix—my sign that I am about to begin pushing. Over to the mattress I moved – quiet, not a word spoken, no sound, intense focus, my eyes drifted closed as I visualized my surrounds and the birth passage of this child. I picture a rose bud opening in a sea of stars, the universe as the back drop. Two deep pushes and the baby was out, born at 8:00 am on the 30th October, a five-hour birth journey, with only myself, my husband and our colleague. Our midwife was not there. His name … Rui.

Anais' birth

It was Monday night 11th December, 2006. All was very calm outside. The night was a little chilly but not cold or storming. Everything about this pregnancy and birth had been different. From the five pregnancy tests to confirm my inner knowing, to ignoring the dot on the mid thigh of my left leg because I didn't want to think I could be pregnant again. We had always wanted to have three children. But so soon?

This baby, like Anam, its eldest brother, was returning 'a positive' when asked if I was carrying twins. I intuitively felt that I was carrying only one. Knowing that nothing is ever missing, it simply is in another form, I thought perhaps my book I was writing at the time, *The Vital Truth: Accessing the possibilities of unlimited health*®, was the twin. Both were to be 'birthed' at a similar time and one had a very blue cover!

This pregnancy and birth was all about position. During the pregnancy I was continuing to write my book and there were times during which I was made to take a position, a stance on what it was I was attempting to convey to the audience. We were also renovating our house at the time so we were living in different 'positions', my husband changed his 'position' at work and our children took to new positions in the family as they each reached their own independent milestones. This baby was taking a stance as well … in a breech position.

It was at five months that I intuitively knew that something was different. We were in Fiji, one last trip away as a family of four and before we returned home to start project managing the renovations on the house. In Fiji, while lying on a deck chair looking out to sea, I said to Randall 'this one's different, it's breech.' Randall smiled and said, 'There is plenty of time for this one to turn.' I smiled back and we didn't really converse about it again; we were busy focusing on the boys and the experience we were all having. I hadn't told anyone about the breech position because I didn't want anyone telling me I was crazy, stupid, or an irresponsible parent, nor did I want to be told that I needed to be in hospital or at the very least should consider a C section if *you want your baby born alive*. Drama, drama, drama. I didn't want the unsolicited information that I knew I would get when telling people, much like the person in the Hy-Vee supermarket saying 'When it all slows down honey … take the drugs!' I absolutely backed myself 100% and knew that the baby would be born safely, at home in beautiful surrounds. The twins had taught me to back myself, to trust in my body's ability 100% and to trust 100% in the unborn child too. Trust I did.

When we moved back into the house after the renovations I started to constantly feel these flutters down low, like wiggling feet. I kept saying to Randall 'this baby is breech'. At one stage Randall did a very specific, very gentle external rotation and it was like adjusting concrete. I knocked his hands away and said 'stop ... this baby and I have chosen this position as the best position for us to birth in. I trust that knowing.' Randall was fine with whatever I decided, after all it was my body and he knew if I truly didn't believe I could do this I wouldn't be in this position. He gave me immense encouragement and support.

My whispers at the beginning of this pregnancy said *'this will be a text book birth. Document it, record it for all to share. This birth will have a special educational ramification and go out on the communication highway.'* I trusted what I heard and wrote it down.

Monday night 11th December, 2006

8:36 pm: I hadn't read anything while pregnant with the boys, nor had we entered into the allopathic 'system' of birth. We always had associated with the pregnancy a midwife or four—our Amish 'mothers'. However before I went to bed this night I came across a wonderful breech website and started reading. Some of the stories had women mentioning hospital and I stopped reading those ones straight away. I didn't need to read about the drama of hospitals and other people telling you what to do. We had always envisaged a home birth and I was prepared for that situation. I read a story of a lady who had a breech birth for her fourth child born at home with a midwife called Sarah. Her story was beautiful and her birth fast, a mere forty-five minutes. I heard a faint whisper say to me *one hour and forty minutes*. I was also told *three hours*. After reading the story of this lady I felt this overwhelming sense of readiness. I felt calm, centered and balanced, something I had not felt in my body for many months.

8:45 pm: I closed my computer and, standing up to lean across the desk to close the windows in my study before heading to bed, I suddenly felt quite incontinent. I walked to my husband who was in the next room and said 'Either my waters have broken or I am suddenly incontinent!' I went to the toilet and urinated and then went down stairs to shower … there was so much 'wee'.

8:50 pm: While in the shower I felt my vagina and realised that it was indeed my waters that had broken. When I got out of the shower I was dripping on the bathmat and I thought I saw some blood but you had to look really closely to notice. I then urinated again and had a mild bloody show. I never had that with the boys so this too was a new experience. I dried myself and went to lie down in bed. I said to Randall, 'It shall be any time.'

9:18 pm: I had my first contraction. I knew it was going to happen tonight and asked Randall to turn off my bedside light in anticipation of getting some rest. He came around and turned off the light and he left the room. As he left the room the light turned back on. I was initially shocked but then a delightful smile came across my face, a knowing. I thought about the vision I had back in March when we conceived this child. Two weeks before making love I was given a name 'Orlando'. 'Orlando … really?' I'd say to myself. I didn't realise the significance of it until later in the pregnancy and certainly now upon reflection. Orlando means 'bright light'. I lay there marveling at the connectedness of this child I was carrying and about to birth. I felt the contractions become more intense and regular. I wanted to stay lying down to slow the process down, to enjoy this moment, my last moment of pregnancy and birth however my intuition was telling me to stand up and walk around.

10:00 pm: We were going to just have two colleagues and ourselves, one to help with the birth due to my birthing position and the other to attend to the needs of the boys. However when we shared that the baby was in a breech position about four weeks before we were going to birth some orange flags went up and they asked if we could coordinate a midwife for the birth. We rang the midwife we used for Rui, our second son's birth, the one who ended up not being present. Ironically I didn't see her at this birth either; she wasn't available. However I did see the other lady who worked alongside her and she was available. She told me she had only been at one home breech birth before and I said 'Well, it's one more than me so come along. Oh, and if you have any other midwives in training than bring them too, if this can help them with other women than I'm okay to have them come.' Again, this birth and pregnancy showed signs of being different; in the past I would never have said yes to anyone coming to the birth—it's just not who I am.

It felt right having somebody at the birth whom I had not meet before. I continued to stay in the bedroom, walking and stopping, leaning on the dressing table when the contractions were present. I kept saying to myself in my mind *each contraction brings me one closer to meeting our baby.* Being a very visual person, I had felt frustrated during the pregnancy because I couldn't get a visual of the birth. With the boys there were many whispers that I listened to. However with this baby the whispers were different ... *12th December ... midnight (I'd had the day and morning birth experience) ... at home ... near the spa in our bedroom ... length of time ... three hours ... with one hour forty minutes of active labour.*

In hindsight I know why I wasn't given a person visual. I would have been irritated knowing somebody who I didn't know would be present and also that eight people would be in the room … watching!

11:30 pm: The contractions were intensifying, however I was still having a reasonable break to sit, breath, chat and smile between them. Mind you, all the Braxton hicks I had been having over the past two months were now serving me well. I started to feel a little anxious at the thought of not knowing what a breech birth would 'be' like however I never wavered in my focus.

11:59 pm: I went around to my side of the bed to look at the time. The contractions started in earnest and I felt the need to go to the toilet. While on the toilet I was reminded of the cry I had had the previous Sunday in the early hours of the morning. I wasn't sure why, I just needed to cry. I went out to the lounge room so as not to wake Randall and cried and cried. I was asking myself all kinds of questions; angry, impatient. I suddenly felt a presence in the room. Sitting on the chair next to me was a friend who had past away the previous Sunday. I stared at what most would think was a vacant chair … she said 'Sare it's just about love and patience.' I cried and cried some more and repeated to myself over and over 'it's just about love and patience.' The tears wouldn't stop at this point and I had been going for about an hour already. As I retraced the previous Sunday night in my head I removed my watch; present now to enjoy the journey, the experience and the outcome. There was no hurry; I was free of time restraints. As I placed my watch on the bedside table the time said 11:59pm. 'Ok, anytime from now is perfect.' In one minute it would be the 12th December.

By now all the members of 'the team' were present in the house. I was in our bedroom so I could pace the flow of people—careful not to overwhelm myself visually. I had always thought I would be on my own for a large portion of the birth journey, and I was. Randall was running in and out making sure everyone was taken care of, not just me!

When one of the contractions had subsided I turned to Randall and asked for our colleague. I wanted a neuro-emotional adjustment, like I had with Rui's birth, to raise my awareness as to what was happening with my thought process. As our colleague came in I immediately started crying on his shoulder 'I don't know if I can do it'. Randall and our colleague from Rui's birth both know that when I get to this stage I am very close to transition and a baby in my arms. He ran an NET on just that: my thought of 'I don't know if I can do it' and immediately in connecting with the thought I was in transition—vomiting and gagging again being my key indicators.

We ran another NET on the baby. He adjusted me and then I called for Randall, who was right beside me anyway; I didn't know as my eyes were closed. The call was the sign that we are ready to push. Randall and I assumed our positions: him holding me up, his arms wrapped around my chest as I stand with my arms around his neck. My head turned to the right, my left cheek and ear over his heart. As I began to push I felt a burning sensation stronger than I recall having with the vertex birth of the boys. I pushed again. Slowly, with each push, my head turned further to the front, my chin now firmly planted into Randall's sternum as I pushed again. My head began to arch backwards as I pushed more. The feet were out and so was one of the shoulders. The midwife was holding the baby's feet, giving it support.

As my head was flexed all the way backwards I remembered being told by my father-in-law, the late Dr Graham Farrant MD, that the position the mother is in during birth is the position that the baby is in. At that moment I saw the baby 'stuck' with their chin on my pubic bone, head arched all the way back which at times can be one of the challenges with a breech birth. I focused on the baby and moving together; mirroring. I very slowly, but very confidently began to tuck my chin and slowly pull it backwards with my forehead moving towards Randall's chest. It wasn't until my chin was tucked in so tight that I felt the need to push again ... one push ... and the baby was birthed.

12:28 pm: A beautiful baby girl, Anais, born breech and unassisted. She had done so very well. She is the 'bright light' in our life. When we had conceived her I was given a vision of a heart beating. I saw it consistently. My friend who had passed away certainly helped me to integrate it all when she said 'it's just about love and patience.'

Anais was born on the 12th December, 2006, 7lbs 4oz. Her birth day in the book of birthdays says the 12th of December is 'The day of taking a stance.' How befitting that she was breech. There are no mistakes in the journey of life.

I breastfeed all our children up until about two years, give or take a couple of months either side. I was either pregnant and breastfeeding or breastfeeding for what seemed like an eternity. The day after Anais' birth I was sitting in the arm chair out in our lounge room breastfeeding her, Rui was fast asleep and Anam quietly walked up behind me so as not to startle her. He came to my right side, the side she was feeding on. He paused, looking at her feeding and then kissed her forehead—softly, tenderly. And with absolute certainty in his voice and knowing in his eyes looked at me and said 'Mum, this is the girl who died when I was born.' I smiled and a tear ran down my cheek. 'I believe you,' I said with a quivering chin. My twins were with me after all, they chose to separate their journey. Unaware at the time I called one Anam and the other Anais as any mother of twins would do, affording them similar names.

I had come full circle with my children, *all my children*, and what a journey thus far it has been.

 Ah ha!

* Find a midwife/birthing partner who you trust to sit at your feet during your child's birth.

* You and your partner have nine months to get used to a home birth idea. Don't compromise on your place of birth.

* Observe the beautiful, innate ways of the body—both of yours and your child's—during your pregnancy and birthing process.

Conclusion

'He who thinks he can and he who thinks he cannot are both right.'

— Henry Ford

When my blinkers were on I thought health was about feelings, food and fitness … period. If your body looked and felt taut, tight and terrific and no signs or symptoms where present then, according to my world and the books I read, you were 'healthy'. How naïve I was. I was led to believe for the first ten years of my life via the language used by my mother, the deliberate actions she took and my observations of these that health was given to me by something and/or someone other than myself. Indeed, I was taught that health was given to me from the outside-in by things I consumed (medications) or things I did (physical fitness, eating good food, positive thoughts and being in a happy state) all of which determined my level and expression of health.

Back then I was medically compliant, dutifully taking what was given to me without question somewhat like Pavlov's dog and his experiment on classical conditioning. There was a medical obedience within myself, my family and amongst my friends I hung out with and the other families we mixed with too. There was a mantra repeated over and over … 'What, you're sick? Well, you had better get something for it.' When 'it' (the symptom) wasn't there anymore then people, parents, peers and the private school I attended deemed me to be healthy once again.

Interesting, isn't?

Right now, in the palm of your hand you have choice either do something different or stay where you are. In other words you can live an illusion that health is given to you by something or someone other than yourself and continue to do the same health approach over and over again, expecting a different result which may or may not ever come—which is the definition of insanity —*or* you can pause … for a moment … the next time you create a health expression and quieten the noise within your head and the need *do it the way it has always been done.*

After all, that is how it all came about for me.

If you remember I was in mum's car looking out the window whilst she was in getting my amoxicillin prescription fulfilled … I paused and searched within myself for a way to approach my health differently. The understanding of nerve system integrity or my recent definition of health was not in my life then. But a seed my dad had planted three years prior was. For the first time in my short life I drew on knowledge I had learnt which was different to what everybody else was doing and mustered *the confidence and the courage* to go against the grain and refuse a medication offered to me by my mum. I was ten years old and haven't looked back.

It is my wish that the knowledge contained within this life-changing book will be yours to germinate in the way you see fit.

You've been given organised vital health information and access to resources to gain the confidence to go against what everybody else is doing. Once the illusionary health bubble is burst, medical obedience halted, the indoctrinated system imploded and your understanding of health and the human body expanded, you WILL begin to express health differently.

I hope that in *'organising the world's health information into bite-sized pieces so people can understand it'* you—as one of those people—have been inspired to slowly but surely take the steps to approaching health from a different perspective.

At the start of this book I spoke about everything not being as it may seem. People's lives are being changed every day by the choices they make or don't make. **The Buddhists say *we'll teach them the illusion until they are ready for the truth.* People are consistently being conditioned to ask the wrong question within an establishment that than doesn't have to TELL YOU THE TRUTH.** Not until you take the time to reframe your view on health and question what is truth will you 'see' an establishment accountable for the lives of the elderly, adults, teenagers, tweens, children, toddlers, babies and infants—lost and never to be returned—simply because of how people are choosing to approach health and not question *the way it has always been done.*

If you *believe* you cannot live a life without medications, then you are right. However **I'm here as testament to a belief that you *can live a life without medications* and so, too, are Randall, Anam, Rui and Anais.**

There is a catalyst for change in every family ... will you be the catalyst in yours?

Ah ha!

* Are you ready to take responsibility for learning which
  health approaches are best for you and your family, and
  to explore the philosophy of each?

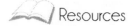 Resources

'I'm doing this for the rest of my life.. will you?'
www.VitalMoms.com/healthillusion

Vital Moms
The **MOST INCREDIBLE** Free Gift **EVER**

How To Claim Your <u>$633.91</u> Worth of Healthy Information

Gift #1: Audio MP3: 'What you don't know can hurt you and your children!'

Gift #2: Monthly Ezine: *Vital Communications* tips for living a vital family life

Gift #3: Chapter Resources:
    Chapter 4: 'Fevers: don't use Paracetamol'
    Chapter 5: 'The bully or the bullied'
    Chapter 8: 'Got a cut lick your wound'
    Chapter 9: 'The magnificent you'
    Chapter 10: 'Health approach quick reference guide'
    Chapter 14: 'Lying lexicon'
    Chapter 16: 'The significance of the wibbly tooth'
    Conclusion: 'I'm doing this for the rest of my life…will you?'

BONUS: Opportunity for a Vital Health Momentum Session with Dr Sarah or one of our Vital Moms coaches

To claim your free Vital Moms gifts go here:
<u>www.VitalMoms.com/healthillusion</u>

OR

Go straight to the Vital Moms club here:
<u>www.VitalMoms.com/club</u>

About the Author

Dr Sarah Farrant, DC is a global selling and award-winning author of *The Vital Truth*[R] and a 'tell it like it is', no fluff, mentor to mums. She is the founder of <u>www.VitalMoms.com</u> *the #1 place for smart health choices for your family!* Dr Sarah's goal in establishing Vital Moms was simple 'to organise the world's health information into bite-sized pieces so people can understand it.' Today she 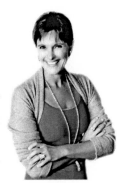 supports, mentors, and educates thousands of people globally . Vital Moms is dedicated to helping parents move away from the 'treatment merry-go-round' by giving them a new way to view and approach their own and their children's health. Dr Sarah has authored books, e-books, reports, articles and been interviewed on radio, TV and by numerous print media. She has three children—all home birthed, non-medicated and now home educated!

Here are some ways to stay connected …

Sample platter: Register for a complimentary copy of our monthly ezine 'Vital Communications'

Select a few: Download our additional and FREE resources <u>www.VitalMoms.com/healthillusion</u>

Hone in: Become a Vital Moms club member at <u>www.VitalMoms.com/club</u>

Deep dive: Attend an event in either the UK, Europe, Middle East, NZ, USA, or Australia. For more information about events, see <u>www.vitalmoms.com/mediapr.</u>

Notes

1. Adapted from http://www.sciencekids.co.nz/sciencefacts/humanbody/nervoussystem.html

2. American College of Preventative Medicine. 'Over the counter medications: use in general and special populations, therapeutic errors, misuse, storage and disposal.' [Online] 2011. [Cited: 22 Mar 2012.]

3. http://www.acpm.org/resource/resmgr/timetools-files/otcmedstimetool.pdf

4. http://www.etymonline.com/index.php?allowed_in_frame=0&search=pathic&searchmode=none

5. http://www.etymonline.com/index.php?allowed_in_frame=0&search=alternative&searchmode=none

6. http://www.etymonline.com/index.php?allowed_in_frame=0&search=alternate&searchmode=none

Index